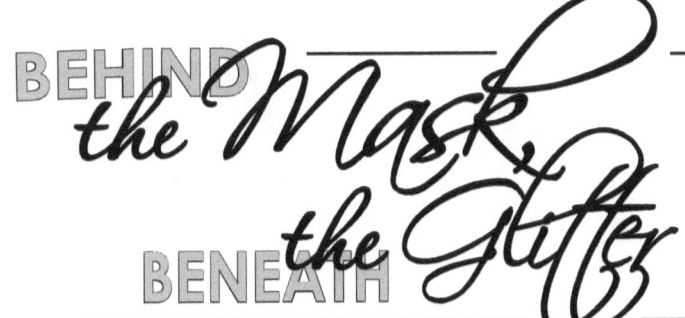

BEHIND the Mask, BENEATH the Glitter

The Deeper Truths about Safe, Smart Cosmetic Surgery

by
Robin T.W. Yuan, M.D.

ISBN: 1451513836
ISBN-13: 9781451513837
LCCN: 2010909864

For autographed or hard cover copies: email request to
robinpbhps@aol.com

DEDICATION

* * *

*To mentors and patients who have taught me
the intricacies and joys of my profession*

TABLE OF CONTENTS

* * *

PREFACE

* * *

Cosmetic surgery is so interesting. It is common and public, yet private and intimate. It is neither solely medicine and science, nor art and inspiration. It is part business and marketing, and part creativity and humanism. It is full of questions that have no answers and concepts that are malleable. It is as popular a topic as sex and money, and fosters opinions just as diverse.

For more than twenty years now, despite the burgeoning interest in, and attention to, cosmetic surgery by individuals, society, and the media, the same questions from patients keep surfacing. It seems obvious to me that the public has quite persistent misconceptions about the field and, despite the focus on safety, too many patients are still facing avoidable injury and complications.

I want to provide patients and the public with insight that goes deeper than what seems on the surface and to arm them with knowledge that will allow them the great benefits of cosmetic surgery while reducing their risks of dissatisfaction. Besides, it is quite interesting to think about what truths lie under the surface. While I have referred to patients in the text by alternating gender, the truths themselves are not gender-specific but are applicable to all persons.

Robin T.W. Yuan, M.D.
Beverly Hills, California

INTRODUCTION

"Doctor, what do you think I need?"
"What do you think you need?"
"Well, you're the expert!"

* * *

A dear friend of mine, a former television journalist and reporter, whom I have known for my entire professional career, had asked virtually all of the important questions that thousands of patients have asked me at one time or another: How long will a face-lift last? Do you think I need this surgery? What will I look like after the procedure? What would you do if you were me? What's the best procedure at my age? Who's the best surgeon in town?

On every occasion, I exasperated her with an age-old Socratic ploy I learned at Harvard College by answering her with questions of my own: How long do *you* want it to last? Do *you* think you need this? What do *you* want to look like? What do *you* want to do? What do *you* think is the best procedure for you? What do *you* think makes the *best* surgeon?

I could tell that she wanted to kill me. Who wants a doctor who answers your question with a question? What good is a doctor who makes *you* answer the questions you want *him* to answer?

Patients want bottom-line answers. "Just the facts, doc," as Sergeant Friday might say.

The public's impression of cosmetic surgery is shaped by stereotypical presumptions, convenient portrayals in the media, and the influence of ubiquitous marketing. Only after I explained the elements of this book and laid out my philosophy did my friend finally exclaim, "Now I get it!" At long last she understood why I could not give a pat answer to her simple question, "What can you do for me?"

I know she wants me to answer with the specifics and certainty an expert should provide: a little Botox here, a bit of Juvederm there, a browlift with periorbital laser and removal of fat under the eyes, a prejowl implant with submental platysmal tightening and liposuction with fat injections to the lips, Alloderm to the vermillion border, and a lower face and necklift with corset platysmaplasty. You'll look fabulous! Oh, and about your nose...

On the other hand, perhaps she doesn't want to know.

The truth is (and this is what Socrates was after) her question has less to do with me, and all to do with her. What *I can do* is not necessarily what *she wants*. The difficulty for her stems from the multiple misconceptions about this very personal field—misconceptions that are perpetuated by the media and surgeons alike. I sense that intelligent and inquisitive patients like her are unintentionally confused, but also often intention-ally misled. I want them to understand the real under-pinnings of cosmetic plastic surgery. Can I show how they can "get it" by stripping away the façade, the ego, and the hype? Might "getting it" in cosmetic surgery require insight into oneself: a most useful, and diffi-cult, principle for life in general? What is it that a sur-geon *should* do?

Whether my patient is the wife of a successful busi-nessman or herself a successful businesswoman, an at-torney for the County of Los Angeles, a fashionable daughter of a foreign billionaire, or a dedicated pub-lic school teacher, each has an individual life story and how he or she relates to his or her own face or body. She has her questions and personal opinions about what is right or wrong. He has his own culture and values. At the same time, each is looking towards me, the "highly educated expert," for answers.

This is really the first misstep; I believe that the first and foremost element of my expertise is not surgical prowess, learned knowledge, or technological wiz-ardry but, rather, the long-lost art of *listening*. I don't give patients answers. I just help them find the answers themselves.

I have relationships, marriages, and jobs depend on the plastic surgery I do or don't do, although I'm sure some patients will soon forget my name like the fourth boyfriend they dated in college or what they had for lunch two Mondays ago. But the tasks, respon-sibility, and the ordeal I put each of them through are similar, developed over the years through many listen-ing sessions, successful or sometimes not, with many patients and would-be patients. The process can be, even *should* be, unexpectedly challenging in the most positive sense of the word. As in life, it requires communication, compromise, and mutual commitment to avoid the innumerable potential disasters along the way. Ultimately, the time spent preparing for surgery can greatly exceed the time spent in surgery. But it is well worth it.

The longer I've cared for patients and the more repetitive the relentless questions, the more I believe **truisms**—*really truthful answers*—are needed, shed of the hype, the salesmanship, the glamour, the glitz, and the ego. And not just pre-programmed, politically correct, five-second sound bite, Google-easy answers.

The fascination and philosophical basis for me derive from the premise—the undeniable truth—that what patients do in cosmetic plastic surgery is unnecessary. Let me repeat because this is important—*really important*—and an extraordinarily odd thing for a plastic surgeon to say: ***Cosmetic surgery is unnecessary***.

Having heard that, and intuitively knowing it is the truth, many people still look at me in disbelief as if I were cutting my own throat. Perhaps I am. But being unnecessary doesn't mean unimportant, meaningless, or without value or consequences. It is still *serious* stuff. It certainly isn't frivolous; a person's health and self-esteem are on the line. As said to Peter Parker (a.k.a. Spiderman) and by President Franklin Delano Roosevelt, with this great power to affect people's lives comes great responsibility. Asking for "unnecessary" surgery changes everything about what to do and how to do it; that is where the process for the patient begins.

While cosmetic surgery is wildly popular in our society and culture (particularly in Beverly Hills and even more so in certain countries like Brazil and

Argentina), it is still about an individual. It is about who the individual is and what he or she wants. I don't operate on a society or a culture or a trend or on a statistic, although all of these things influence patients. **I operate on individuals.**

While I strive to listen to you and learn about you, I am not you. I am not the expert of your life and your body. You are.

I am constantly on the lookout for truisms, even if they are contrary to conventional beliefs and not the things that patients want to hear. It is especially important if I get patients to *think* and help to integrate all that goes on in cosmetic surgery with their life in general. Procedures I am doing today are not the procedures I did five years ago and won't be the procedures I will do in another five years. But hopefully the truths that I discuss and expose beneath the veneer are immutable and unassailable, and will be just as applicable when I retire.

Early in my career, an internist sent me her patients for consultation. I gave them an honest assessment. Later, I heard that she told a mutual friend, in jest I think, that she should stop referring to me. She said I kept telling her patients they didn't need surgery: she was sending me bread and butter patients, and I was sending them home. I was pretty proud of that. It was a truism; cosmetic surgery is not a necessity. This internist couldn't believe a Beverly Hills plastic surgeon would send patients home without signing them up for a procedure. The irony is that this doctor's patients still seek me out despite what I tell them because they appreciate honesty more than they value pat answers, and while sitting at home, they often discover that they really do *desire* the surgeries I offer. Many of them have become my most loyal patients.

* * *

So here it is, the result of my search for truth, the goal of which is to allow readers, prospective patients or not, a framework and foundation to examine their own lives and the truths about cosmetic surgery. Could it be that in peeling back the layers of hype, cutting through the sheen of all that glitters, and peeking behind the inscrutable surgeon's mask, that in searching for meaning in seemingly unnecessary cosmetic surgery, you can find the meaning to life itself? Perhaps not. But finding some meaning and priorities, the *desires,* in your own individual life may be quite possible, even necessary.

There is very little in this book that involves specific techniques, how-I-do-it procedures, or recipes for beauty enhancement from the rich and famous who dart in and out of the many medical offices in Beverly Hills; those are constantly changing. You will not find instructions on how to care for yourself after a laser face peel, information on what types of anesthesia are available for facelifts, what the post-operative recovery is like following an abdominoplasty, or how to finance your breast implant surgery. Those are easy questions to answer; your surgeon will do it for you. Rather, I strive to reveal some of the inside-the-mind machinations derived from a *philosophical* approach to cosmetic surgery. These are what inherently drive the practical workings of the profession and lead to the *decision* for that same laser face peel, facelift, or abdominoplasty. By integrating elements of cosmetic surgery with other facets of life, *truisms*, often contrarian and surprising, are revealed.

Cosmetic surgery does not exist in a vacuum. It mirrors life and life mimics it. In clinical medicine, we have a saying based on Ockham's razor learned early in medical school: "When you hear hoof beats, think horses, not zebras"; that is, think of the *common, not the rare*. But I prefer to paraphrase: When you hear hoof beats, *only* if you are sure it is *not* a zebra can you assume that it's probably a horse; in life, the obvious is obvious, but the obscure is not. Like investments, when everyone is chasing something, it's often time to look in the opposite direction. Doctors do not like to miss the obvious, but they revel even more in uncovering the obscure. Likewise, patients need not follow the stampeding crowd. They need to define their own individual stripes.

There are no easy assumptions in the field of cosmetic surgery. A patient's fervent and wholly common belief to the contrary, my listening experience, a healthy dose of skepticism, and an affinity for the truth lead me to realize that there is no such thing as 'best' in cosmetic surgery. Likewise, a whole album of before-and-after photos might not tell you much, and you really can't predict what reward or result you are going to get until you actually get it. There are few absolute "knowns" in cosmetic surgery. Such are the revelations.

Not all questions have neat little answers that I can provide in a five-minute consultation, and not all cosmetic problems have sound surgical solutions; *easy answers are not always the right answers*. This presents a real quandary. Patients, like my longtime friend, demand definitive answers for their desires and expectations, and they want it quick. They don't expect to be pressed with soul-searching questions that might take weeks, months, or a lifetime to digest. The business and marketing of cosmetic surgery, while feeling very foreign and out-of-place in the hallowed halls of serious, life-saving medicine, need to project unequivocal solutions, predictable results, and concrete and effective products like the marketing of Dell computers.

The traditional goals of keeping a patient well, at home, and out of the hospital are turned on their collective heads by the practical necessity of getting a prospective patient motivated to act on her desires. She is persuaded to purchase an admission ticket into the magical kingdom of surgical enhancement, and, eventually after the dust settles, to feel more attractive, more energetic, more self-confident, more whatever it is she wants. Plastic surgeons are faced with the enviable luxury of operating on relatively normal, healthy people. In exchange for that luxury, we are tasked by a rather unenviable challenge: making a *well* patient *"more well."* How *do* we do that?

It all depends, of course, on what a patient *means* by "more well," how she *communicates*, how her surgeon *interprets* what he hears…or if the surgeon *listens* at all.

* * *

Recently, one of my patients called my office. She had had a breast augmentation and lift over two years prior. Doctors, being generally defensive, cautious, and a bit paranoid, face such out-of-the-blue calls from former breast patients with dread because we fear a complication has occurred or disenchantment with the surgical results has set in. This patient had just seen an episode of a nationally televised talk show following the very public post-operative death of a popular singer's mother. The show focused on plastic surgery gone wrong. I hadn't seen the program but I imagined all the horror stories.

Did her implants "explode"? Were her nipples purple? Had she been diagnosed with cancer? Was I going to get an earful of what was disappointing to her? Did all the questions she asked and all the answers I made her give me dredge up some deep-seated discontent? Could I have missed something in her history? Did something horrible happen to her over the last two years that she was hiding from me, and did the television show give her courage to confront me? My whole career flashed before my eyes with this call.

"I was sitting there watching the show, Dr. Yuan." *Uh-oh*, I thought, expecting the worst. "And I realized how lucky I was to have you as my doctor."

I relaxed a bit as I furiously scanned her chart, looking for signs as to what was coming next, still not knowing why she was calling. The chart offered no clues.

"Some patients on the show saw their doctor for only five minutes, or not at all," she continued. "They talked to some assistant! Some cosmetic doctors weren't even trained! And operating in a strip mall?" She paused. I didn't know if she was getting emotional or had paused for dramatic effect. "I wanted you to know how much I appreciated the ordeal" (did she really say "ordeal"?), "the many hours of consultation you put me through before surgery, the thought that went into my surgery, the hands-on post-op care. My boyfriend and I are so *very* happy with everything. I was blessed!"

I felt a calm come over me. Knowledge, safety, happiness—that's what it's all about.

"You *need* to know how much I appreciate you, Dr. Yuan." She stressed the *need*.

Truth. She "got it." It nearly made me cry.

With that, let's begin.

CHAPTER 1:

COSMETIC SURGERY IS UNNECESSARY

* * *

The patient sits nervously in an easy chair in the office. She is studying a dozen diplomas hanging on the wall like big game trophies: one from Harvard University, one from Harvard Medical School, four from surgical residency programs in Los Angeles and Miami, an American Board of Plastic Surgery certificate, memberships in numerous professional societies, and a handful of Who's Who plaques. There are photos of the plastic surgeon with celebrity-patients, world famous musicians, distinguished mentors, a Nobel laureate, and notable surgeons from around the globe. The patient has mustered the courage and has allotted what she hopes will be adequate finances, and now awaits recommendations for her cosmetic concerns. She has been referred to the surgeon by a variety of well-respected sources: her gynecologist, a general surgeon, her internist, her best friend, and a neighbor, perhaps even her hairstylist. It is with a common mixture of anxiety and excitement, embarrassment and determination, fear and desire that the patient anticipates the plastic surgeon's arrival.

Just as the possibility of getting up out of the chair and escaping the inner sanctum enters the patient's mind, the surgeon walks in, exchanges pleasantries, and asks the patient what he can do to help her. As the patient self-consciously describes what bothers her, the plastic surgeon listens intently. The patient starts slowly, gradually warming to him. He nods with understanding and interest, silently encouraging her personal exposition. More of her life spills out into the room. She gains confidence and talks of her job, her family, and her education. She explains her history of weight loss and weight gain, the pregnancies, her diet, and exercise routine. She touches on her childhood, how she felt growing up. She can't believe she is telling him so much. Fifteen minutes have gone by and he has barely uttered a sentence.

When finished, the patient boldly inquires, "What do you think? What do I need?"

The plastic surgeon leans back in his leather chair. With all of the diplomas, he must be smart. She thinks he looks honest. He has wisps of white at his temples. That must mean he has some experience. He has done thousands of operations and is touted to be "one of the best," if not "THE BEST," plastic surgeon in the city (an impossible appellation, as we shall later see). She might have seen a number of other plastic surgeons but is still looking for answers that will satisfy her.

She sees him look her straight in the eye, and he gives the answer she was *not* looking for, is *least* expecting, but *cannot* dispute.

"Cosmetic surgery is *unnecessary*..."

The plastic surgeon pauses, looking for some reaction. He is not disappointed. The patient is stunned. *What is he talking about? No one else has said this. Am I in the wrong office? What plastic surgeon would admit that what he does is unnecessary? Is he turning away my business? Does he think I am beyond help? Does he think I am crazy?*

Now, she is feeling embarrassed. *I shouldn't be here,* she thinks. *This was a foolish idea. This doctor's a fool... he's condescending, he's self-righteous, he's mocking me. And yet...he is right.* Plastic surgery, that is, *elective, cosmetic* plastic surgery, *is* unnecessary.

"But..." the plastic surgeon is finishing his thought, "it is *desirable.*"

Ahhhhhh. Yes. That's better. It is desirable because I desire it. It is okay to want what this fool can provide. The patient nods, thinking to herself, *I get it. Unnecessary, but desirable. Want, not need. He isn't a fool. Maybe he is just being honest.*

The plastic surgeon sees the recognition of truth that nearly all patients sitting in the easy chair display as the muscles in the patient's face react. The brows relax. The smile returns. He nods in empathy for her feelings about herself and her understanding of what just took place. It is not a gesture of pity. It is, perhaps, the beginning of an epiphany.

* * *

A variation of this little scene is played out with every cosmetic surgery patient in my office, be it a young female looking for a shapelier nose, a maternal woman desiring smaller, uplifted breasts, a mother seeking a postpartum sculpting of her newborn's unexpected gift, or a middle-aged divorcee hoping to put forth a more youthful face for the world to see. The play can involve husbands, boyfriends, or even children who weave in and out of the plot, as well as in and out of the consultation room. Sometimes it is a one-act play—straight to the point—in a very assertive and mature life. Other times it is a complex three-act play with marriages, affairs, teenage angst, financial woes, and deaths as subplots. Occasionally it is an endless drama perpetuated by insecurities, indecision, and inner conflicts.

The motivation for cosmetic change is driven not by procedures nor techniques nor machines nor medicines and, especially, should not be compelled by me or any other plastic surgeons with all of our diplomas, certificates, and training. But ultimately, and ideally (and this may take a lifetime), it is a search for truth—the truth about the patient's self and what each individual desires. There is a reason each patient sits in that easy chair and why it really is an *uneasy* chair. There is something that each person wants and the mere act of sitting in that chair can be a significant step toward discovery.

So you might think, *I don't* need *to be here...*

But you are.

I do not take lightly the fact that a patient is physically sitting in front of me. Yes, it is what I *want* and what I *expect*, and, if I am responsible for feeding my family as well as my ego, what I *need*. Every plastic surgeon feels the same way. It is so automatic and mindless to expect. In fact, we are disappointed when patients don't show up; when they cancel, it is like being stood up on your first date. But in today's world of easy, non-stop information and Internet access, home-delivered food, instantaneous text messaging, and cellular phone communications at the speed of light, the actual process of arriving at my doorstep can be a tedious, self-effacing, introspective, traffic-impeded, even depressing journey. Or it can be a whim—a what-the-hell, spur-of-the-moment, impulsive act. I do not know. But I appreciate the fact that a patient might have had to face a number of demons and obstacles, both physical and emotional, to get to the point of picking up the phone and doing all the things necessary to get to sit in the uneasy chair in front of me.

She comes with insecurities, discontentment, embarrassment, perhaps even disgust and prodding from others. She has expectations, hopes, imagination, innate trust (maybe distrusts), and desires. What she seeks is truth from me, her plastic surgeon, but also, conscious or not, she is in pursuit of truth about herself. And she'll circle the block three times looking for a parking space to get it.

* * *

Truth. What *is* the truth? What do we mean by truth? Why—and *how*—can some people spend a lifetime chasing it, often without success? Something that is so self-evident is yet so deceptively elusive. Something that is so concrete and seemingly simple—the truth, the whole truth, and nothing but the truth—is often unknown and intangible. It is fact. It is reality. It is the absence of falsehood. It is something that can be proved or verified. But it is also something one may not believe or recognize when it is there.

The patient is searching for her own true self and, in doing so, is making a statement about how she really feels about herself. That seems deep—*too deep*—for plastic surgery. It is too transcendental, too self-revelatory, too New Age. Plastic surgery is supposed to be superficial and frivolous. Go in, get zapped, lifted, suctioned, injected, and "voilá!" you're glamorous, sexy, and happy! Isn't *that* the truth?

While the search may involve a rejection of a patient's reality, as in certain self-loathing body dysmorphism syndromes, it can also be an enlightening, fully self-discovering journey. But the real truth is that very few patients enter the plastic surgeon's office with this quest consciously on their mind. They just want the bump on their nose gone or that bulge on their stomach smaller or their breasts to be a different size or shape. The real reason they are sitting in the chair may be hidden. But being less than conscious about it doesn't mean it doesn't exist. Not being aware of it doesn't mean you shouldn't look for it. There usually is a reason "why" they want the bump removed, the bulge gone, the breasts a different size or shape. At some point, you will need to answer this question of "why?"

The odd thing is that many patients will look at me skeptically when I ask "why?" It is almost as if it is a given that everyone should want whatever it is they want when they want it. They might feel some guilt but they assume that a nose without a bump is better than a nose with a bump or that bigger breasts are better than smaller breasts, or vice versa, as the case may be. Patients don't expect that a plastic surgeon will even be concerned about *why* they want cosmetic surgery. I suppose I shouldn't fault them since it is like a waiter asking a diner why he wants something to eat, or why he is eating in this particular establishment, or why he wants a certain type of food. A waiter doesn't care *why* you want to eat—only *what* you want to eat. He can answer how it is cooked but not why you should eat it. "Why" can sound intimidating, a challenge. And it is. People reveal themselves when put on the spot. It is here where the practicalities of performing cosmetic surgery can bring out an individual's psychology.

The "why" can be related to a feeling the patient had when embarrassed about a "deformity." This is common in males who have gynecomastia, or feminization of the breast, or who were obese as teenagers and thus feel self-conscious about their physique even years later. It can have something to do with looking like someone else, particularly when a woman starts to age and begins to look like her mother; perhaps it would be instructive to see what the mother looks like. Sometimes it has to do with an image of someone that she wants to emulate, perhaps a celebrity, or an idealization of who she thinks she really is. It might be the feeling of defeat when her flesh hangs over the waist when she sits at the dinner table. At other times, it may be a more practical reason, such as being able to wear certain types or sizes of clothing, or maintaining competitiveness in the job market, or giving her a final shot at finding a spouse...for the second, third, or even fourth time. But if you don't know what the "why" is, you can't be sure you have the answer. *"Why" is necessary for "what."*

Besides the understanding and acceptance that there is a truth and reason as to why the patient is in my office, there is the question of how and when do I know the truth when I see or hear it? How does a patient know whether to trust her doctor? How does a patient make a correct decision for herself and when does she know it has been the right one? How does a patient know surgery is worth it? How does truth affect the practice of cosmetic surgery? The key to answering these questions is in accepting the premise that cosmetic surgery is, indeed, unnecessary. It is not a trivial premise to be seconded by a "yeah, yeah, I know." In practice, all else should flow from the acknowledgement of this primary truth.

* * *

Why is it important to acknowledge and believe in this premise? Why can't we just treat the symptoms: the hump on the nose, the flat chest, the sagging neckline? The answer: because *the doctor-patient relationship and the process of formulating a treatment plan are completely different from the usual encounter with a doctor.*

In most physicians' offices dealing with injury or sickness, the patient is seeking a proclamation: You have such-and-such disease; you need the following diagnostic tests; you need to do this treatment or take that medicine or undergo some therapy to get well, or to become whole, or to be cured. The trip to the doctor's office and the diagnostic plan and treatment remedies are generally looked at as necessary. Some suggestions are met with denial, some with skepticism, some with fear, and some with understanding and enthusiasm. But few are seen as unmitigated *un*truths.

The patient expects the proclamation to be true and honest. In fact, the patient demands and assumes it. This proclamation is not an emotional statement, although it might be delivered or received with emotion. It is usually a statement of fact, or logic, or statistics. "There is a five-year cure rate of ninety-five percent with surgical extirpation." "You need to take this antibiotic that is ninety-nine percent effective against the bacteria causing the infection." "We need to do an amputation because the leg cannot be saved." "You require an angiogram and have to cut down on the fat in your diet or you'll have a heart attack that can kill you."

The patient's own opinion may enter the mix but there is no refuting the importance of the doctor's proclamation, even if it is really only his opinion. The patient may not always know if the proclamation itself is true, only that the doctor is hopefully honest about it and has her best interest in mind. The doctor becomes the filter, the definer, the repository of truth, and the motivator for action. **The doctor has the facts and the answer.** The patient's opinion is often secondary, although this is less true as the public becomes empowered with knowledge and there is less "informational asymmetry."

Because of this, whether or not the patient believes she has a disease, whether or not she has faith in a medicine, whether or not she desires a particular surgery will not appreciably impact the outcome or the treatment in most medical situations. If you have diabetes and your blood sugar is abnormal, how you *feel* about yourself won't affect the way a diabetic drug you need to take will work. *Believing* you do or do not have diabetes will not change the fact that you do or do not actually have the disease. Whether you are *happy* or *depressed* or *content* won't alter the results of an amputation or kidney transplantation. If you are Christian or Confucian, Chinese or Czech, desire or detest a brain scan, having a brain tumor is pretty much the same for everyone.

Of course, there are some who believe in the power of positive thinking and would argue against the separation of mind and matter; they believe the mind *can* heal. Many will recognize and appreciate the value of patients as partners, as opposed to passive (or reluctant and uncooperative) subjects in achieving a successful outcome. But most of the cards and how they will be played are in the hands of the doctor, science, and the medical establishment. Treatments certainly vary according to diverse parameters, and opinions may differ or prove to be right or wrong, but few patients will dictate their own medical treatment based on what they believe is normal. Would you decide whether or not to treat a blood glucose of one hundred and fifty or a blood pressure of one hundred and fifty over ninety? Would you tell a surgeon whether or how to do a specific operation even though you may have opinions about the surgery itself? Would you tell a doctor what or how medications should be prescribed even though you may have a preference? Would you feel strongly enough to instruct a radiation therapist on what dose, what machine, or what ports to use? How about telling an orthopedic surgeon what prosthetic system to use or an oncologist which combination of chemotherapeutic agents to use? Not many in their right mind will walk away from treatment that could cure them. Patients feel compelled to act because of the doctor's proclamation.

In fact, most patients feel a comfort in trusting their doctor and leaving decisions in their hands. It is pretty much all about what the doctor thinks and does. It is what I call ***paternalistic medicine.*** You do what your father and mother say because you trust them implicitly or you fear what will happen if you don't. This process of decision-making, or lack of decision-making, is quick, easy, and without risk...for the patient. All you have to do is sit back and do what the doctor says. It is because the treatment is necessary, is based on factual data, and is presumably supported by data or experience, no matter what you believe or think. In fact, there is comfort in that.

The opposite is true for cosmetic surgery—at least in the ideal situation—and for the purist. The patient need not listen to the plastic surgeon because nothing is truly wrong. She is not contagious or dying. She is not, or should not be, dysfunctional in society. She is not diseased and her chemistries are not abnormal. She can see, speak, and swallow. She is not writhing on the floor in pain, vomiting up blood, seeing double, or shaking with chills. The reason the cosmetic patient is in my office is because...she *wants* something. There is a perception, whether real or imagined or desired, that something will benefit her and improve her life in a way that is important to her. Every patient that comes in for cosmetic surgery is a normal person. And I tell them exactly that: *You are a normal person.* Simple, basic, truthful. Yet, you are looking for something.

This was not always the case. Back in the golden age of Hollywood, when the major studios were in control of all aspects of an actor's life, it was not uncommon that some were told to get their nose operated on or their breasts enlarged, or risk loss of employment and marketability. It still happens to an extent today.

Well-meaning parents were also just as guilty of putting their teenage daughters through cosmetic surgery. One "celebrity" wrote about the answer her mother gave when she asked her whether she was pretty. "You will be once we get your nose done," her mother reportedly answered. Many teenagers have lived to regret the various procedures their parents "forced" upon them as necessary to make them whole or attractive or acceptable. Even though parents might have their child's best interest in mind, in all of these situations, the perceived necessity of the surgery rendered the actual patients powerless in their decision-making and choice.

While the pressure to look normal, be more attractive, or project youth is significant, in reality, no one needs a hump on the nose removed. It is not going to make her run faster. No one needs his jowls smoothed out. It is not going to make him live longer. No one needs her wrinkles gone. It is not going to make her heart or lungs function better. No one needs C-cup breasts. It won't make the bowels more regular. Yet the cosmetic patient, and I even hesitate to call her a "patient," wants these things. She wants them so much that she acts in exact contradiction to the patient who wants to run *away* from the surgeon who recommends removing her breast to *cure* her of breast cancer, *away* from the gynecologist who suggests taking her uterus out to *relieve* her of chronic pain, and *away* from the otolaryngologist who prescribes extirpating a *deadly* salivary gland tumor, and who will go to the operating room kicking, screaming, and crying.

On the other hand, cosmetic surgery patients *voluntarily* line up and pay significant hard-earned dollars out of their own pockets to *have* surgery they don't need and often against the advice of parents and friends! What a *crazy* thought! It still amazes me.

Whether or not she is aware of it, the patient is seeking, or already knows, truths about herself. She knows she is normal, but she does not feel normal. She knows she is not sick, but wants to be "better." She knows she is relatively happy, but could be happier. While she may seem to be only concerned with the superficialities of her body (the hump, the bulge, the size), she is really saying something about the quality of her life and how she wants to live it. She must know what pain she feels about what she might consider to be an unattractive or aging face. She must know what discomfort she experiences when she bares her "imperfect" torso. She must anticipate the self-confidence she has to gain with "better-looking" breasts or "shapelier" lips. She must fear her mortality or vulnerability when she points out her wrinkles and sagging skin. She is distinguishing what is meaningful and what is not...for her.

Just like a person who selects a Porsche convertible over a Honda van, a T-bone steak over steamed vegetables, a stately English Tudor over a minimalist condominium, she is exposing her values and tastes, as well as her body. And I, as her plastic surgeon, *must* listen in order to be effective. I must not prejudice myself, no matter how many diplomas I possess, because, as one mature and intelligent patient put it, the truth is that "circumstances (i.e., physical enhancements) that many people say do not make you happy actually have made me *very* happy. And I feel terrific!" It is all about you, the individual patient.

* * *

One of my medical mentors, the surgeon who first exposed me to the wondrous and creative field of plastic surgery, Dr. Joseph Murray, Harvard professor emeritus, gave an illuminating and fervent presidential address to the Boston Surgical Society entitled "Is

Beethoven Necessary?" This was years before he won the Nobel Prize for Physiology or Medicine in 1990 for performing the first successful human kidney transplantation and developing the immunosuppressive drug azathioprine. When I recently communicated with him about this book, he was surprised that I had remembered this rather small and unscientific lecture. Yet it was a seminal event in my career, in part because I was a violinist and a lover of classical, especially Romantic, music.

With this presentation, Dr. Murray eloquently defended the attributes of surgery devoted to physical enhancement. At this time of his life, he was also pioneering the relatively new field of craniofacial surgery that reshaped children's skulls and faces, often producing cosmetic changes motivated by presumed psychosocial, rather than functional, benefit. The talk was given to a group of non-plastic surgery doctors in the hallowed halls of the Harvard Club of Boston, many of whom questioned the value of this burgeoning field of cosmetic surgery, scoffed at plastic surgeons as real doctors, and looked upon cosmetic patients as "frivolous and superficial." Plastic surgery is not about the hump on the nose, the size of the breast, or the shape of the body or head. It is about the patient's soul and self. It is about what makes a human being a human being and not an inanimate object d'art. It is about what gives individuals joy, soothes their pain, and makes their lives more inspired. Without these concerns, human life would be silent, devoid of the *Fifth Symphony, Ode to Joy,* the *Emperor's Concerto,* and my favorite, the *Violin Concerto in D*—all of which are unnecessary to life's basic and rudimentary functions. As I often tell patients, I operate on their faces and bodies, but it is what happens inside their heart and between their ears that is important. Sometimes it works and sometimes it doesn't. But it is what I try to do.

* * *

What does cosmetic plastic surgery have in common with other elements or experiences that are "unnecessary" to human existence? I have often thought that it can be compared to wine. Not everyone will drink it. Some drink it for itself, some for the completeness of the whole meal. There are cheap wines and very expensive ones. Some will think very little of what they drink and others will customize it to their choice of food and individual palates. Most will imbibe responsibly, but some will indulge to the extreme and end up possessed by their very desires. I'll serve it, but I personally don't drink it. It, like most activities in which we engage during life, is unnecessary, even for nourishment. Yet, to many, it is a ubiquitous enhancement to food, the dining experience, and life in general. When it works the way it is supposed to work, it makes you happy.

On the other hand, cosmetic surgery can also seem like a swim in the freezing Atlantic Ocean in the dead of winter. Some find it invigorating and life-enhancing. It risks a chest cold and extreme discomfort, perhaps even frostbite, and it flies in the face of your well-meaning mother's admonishment to dress warmly when going out in the harsh New England climes. Imagine selling pricey tickets to people who want to indulge in this activity. We can either admire their courage and joie de vivre, or we may think that they are quite masochistic, self-destructive, and perhaps crazy.

In addition to the personal and life-enhancing experiences involved in partaking wine or polar dipping in the Atlantic, a cosmetic surgery patient is very conscious of walking away with something tangible. The patient/client/customer is looking for something she wants and can "take home": a busty figure, a clean neckline, and svelte silhouette. As such, she is more like a shopper than a patient. Of primary importance is that she has the luxury of having choices. She can shop wherever she wants and whenever she wants. No one is forcing her, hopefully. She can shop convenience or go boutique. She can go to a volume discount warehouse or a one-of-a-kind chic specialty house. Unlike with medical insurance plans providing for medically necessary care that limit access to doctors or hospitals through contracts or tiered benefits, the cosmetic patient has complete freedom, presumably limited only by her pocketbook.

One can take or leave a Mercedes SL55 convertible, a fifty-two-inch Sony Bravia LCD high-definition television, or a custom-made Vera Wang wedding dress. Plenty of people leave it; not everyone has plastic surgery, even in Beverly Hills. Most live with "imperfections," age gracefully, and marry others, "warts and all." The patient has so much freedom that she doesn't even have to shop. She can choose to say "no." That fact alone makes saying "yes" more significant. It is like answering the question: "Will you marry me?" Not asking the question, not answering it, or saying "no" is relatively easy. Saying "yes" is monumental. It can be life-changing.

There is no denying the availability and the desire for nonessential items. People buy what they want, when they want, to the degree they can afford it. They might listen to a salesman but hopefully they will make their own choice based on their own tastes, expectations, and desires. Some will, and can, buy whatever they want without regard for anyone else's opinion or even in the presence of indisputable facts contradicting their choice. They'll buy a fourth car when they really need only two. They'll buy a piece of art that nobody likes just because it is unusual. They'll dress the way they like despite what anyone else thinks. This becomes the opposite of paternalism. It is completely individualistic and *self*-driven. Unfettered, **self-centered consumerism** is a luxury few can afford and it can be dangerous. It can become chaotic, destructive, and self-indulgent, even as it is empowering, intoxicating, exhilarating, and, thus, addictive.

There are bizarre extremes of cosmetic manipulation bordering on what some might consider self-mutilation rather than self-expression. But it is the force, however small and whether recognized or not, that drives, or should drive, the patient to the plastic surgeon's office. It is all about the patient, and very little about the doctor. It is about what the patient wants, not what the surgeon can do. When shopping for cosmetic surgery, the patient is truly in the driver's seat. It may not seem like it when you first arrive in the room full of diplomas, but you are.

As with most shoppers, especially inexperienced ones, a cosmetic patient may know what she dislikes yet not know exactly want she wants.

"Can I help you?"

"No, thank you. I'm just looking."

Part of the reason is because what she wants is unnecessary. If she needed a specific tool to accomplish a certain task, she would know exactly what to look for. If she were dying of thirst, she'd be looking for water. If her car had a flat tire, she'd be looking for a spare tire or a phone to call a tow truck. If she had a nail to set, she'd be shopping for a hammer. Shopping for necessary items is too easy. One can simply send the spouse.

But shopping for things you desire but do not need forces personal conviction and individuality. It requires effort and commitment, especially if you're on a budget. Just think of how you shop. Do you go straight for the shelf that has what you desire? Do you browse the aisles all befuddled with the variety? Do you tell the sales clerk that you are just looking to get rid of him and buy yourself time? Do you impulsively purchase as soon as you see something or do you go back again and again after looking elsewhere? Do you ask your friends or spouse or parent their opinions or do you prefer to shop solo? Do you listen to advice and opinions or do you ignore them? Do you trust the salesperson and advertisements or are you a skeptic always wary of being "taken"?

There is no single and right way to shop for unnecessary but desirable things. You have to have your own zone of comfort and conviction.

Part of the impediment to knowing what you want is not knowing what is possible. A patient often knows that she is displeased with something or wants to change something but may not know exactly what she wants to end up with; she does not know all the possibilities surgery has to offer.

It is not uncommon for a patient to answer my question, "What do you want?" with "I'm not a doctor. I don't know what you can do." I tell them not to worry about what is possible. That is my responsibility. Just tell me what you want. I am like her surgical concierge. Even then it may take weeks of soul-searching and collaboration in multiple consultations. Just like with forging relationships, a person often can state the type of partner with whom one is *not* compatible (I can't be around cat-lovers because I am allergic to cats) but cannot accurately describe just who *is* their ideal mate. The combination and permutations of possibilities can be paralyzing (just like what I face when in the grocery store choosing cereal for my children, staring at rows of boxes on six shelves, each twenty feet long). In addition, one may even have less of an idea *if* an ideal mate exists.

A cosmetic patient is motivated by some *self*-centered desire. I do not say this in a critical manner but as a matter of fact. It should reflect *his* or *her* desires and please or benefit *his-* or *her*self, not others. My goal, as the plastic surgeon, is to understand the desires and the motivations of the individual patient—*unencumbered by* my own motivations or desires, although not devoid of constraints afforded by experience, knowledge, science, all those diplomas, and also common sense. Plastic surgery thus becomes a blend of paternalism and self-centered medical consumerism. It seems like a logical and practical truism; *let us—you and me—find a solution for you.* Sounds like a commercial for a bank.

CHAPTER 2:

ALL ABOUT YOU

* * *

"**S**o, what do I need, doc?"

I know she is looking to me for answers, for guidance. What she is looking for is fact, but what she is asking for is opinion. I bluntly, although hopefully not disrespectfully, tell the patient that it matters little to me what she wants to look like. It sounds harsh but it soon becomes clear it is rhetorical.

There is no universal beauty. It is not important to *me* if her nose has a bump or not. It is not offensive to *me* that her breasts are as small as apples or as big as melons. It is not important to my life if she has fat under her lower eyelids or jowls along her jaw line. I don't live with her, and I am not married to her. Most people are not Miss Universe and Mr. Adonis. But I don't judge them if they want to attain some of these or any other attributes they desire. It is the patient's prerogative to live life the way she or he wants as long as it doesn't deprive or hurt others.

My main purposes are to keep her safe, interpret her desires, discuss alternatives, and accomplish her anatomic goals as best I can. I am the expressive hand of her artistic desires. She will guide my hand. But she is not entirely alone in her decision-making; she does have me.

It is quite revealing that plastic surgeons do not agree on this concept of collaboration. On many occasions, in private, in meetings, and in discussions in journal publications, plastic surgeons have butt heads over whether surgical decisions and goals should be controlled by the surgeon "because we are the beauty experts," "we know what looks attractive," and "the patient doesn't know, that's why they're here." *Or,* should treatment be dictated by the patient "because it is their body and face" and "who are we to say what a person should or shouldn't look like"? It is almost like religion and evolution. Both sound acceptable, even desirable, within each context. You can easily agree with one or the other concept. You can believe in Christian creationism in Sunday school and Darwinian evolution during final exams. But it is nearly impossible to accept both at the same time.

On one occasion at a local meeting of plastic surgeons in Los Angeles, there was a heated exchange between two surgeons, both of whom specialized in rhinoplasty. Upon being asked by our group to comment on the picture of a third surgeon's potential patient, one of the surgeons began to analyze the nose, critiquing certain contours, angles, and tip projection. He then stated exactly what he would do to perform a beautiful rhinoplasty. One could hardly disagree that the resulting nose would be a structural improvement and satisfy most concepts of what constitutes a classically beautiful nose. It fit the box.

"She needs her hump taken down, her tip thinned, and her nasal bones in-fractured," he said with conviction. We all knew *what* would make the nose more attractive. We had studied classic features of the beautiful nose. For many decades, certainly since the time I began my training, surgeons performed rhinoplasties using the same paradigm for beauty: straight dorsum, narrow bridge, slight rise to a defined tip with well-described angles and effective light reflexes, open angle at the columella-lip junction with narrow, vertically aligned nostrils and gently curved alar rims, and a predetermined projection to length ratio as governed by the Golden Proportion. The only real debate through the years was on *how* to best achieve these aesthetic goals.

The second surgeon asked the question, "What does the patient want?"

The first surgeon replied, "What does it matter what the patient thinks? She doesn't know. That's why she's coming to us. We are the experts! We know proportion and form. We know what looks good."

The room was soon engulfed in an uproar of opinions and disagreements. I could only think about the poor patient. If a small room full of experienced plastic surgeons had such divergent views, whose advice should she follow? What confidence could she have that she had found the truth with any of the answers when it was obvious that not all answers could be correct? Or could they? Where would the truth lie?

I am reminded of a famous story many of my father's neurosurgical colleagues and residents relate about a statement he made to a group of neurologists attending a neuroradiology presentation at a Harvard-affiliated hospital. The neurologists, who are a very brainy and analytical medical breed, were opining about a patient's diagnosis based on signs and symptoms of spinal origin. Upon hearing the many, and opposing, self-assured conjectures, my father boldly proclaimed his most famous quote, "A tube of dye (used in the now-outdated diagnostic myelogram for spinal cord pathology) is worth a roomful of neurologists." The truth lay in the myelogram, not in a room full of opinions. So what is the plastic surgical equivalent of that tube of dye?

A few years later, at a similar meeting of the top plastic surgeons in Los Angeles, a doctor projected a picture of an Asian woman's face on a screen for the other doctors to offer suggestions. The middle-aged woman wanted a more refined nose with a more pronounced bridge. The doctor had placed a silicone implant on her dorsum yet she still wasn't satisfied. He performed another surgery and still she wasn't satisfied. She had a reasonably proportioned, somewhat "Caucasian-looking" nose that seemed a bit "done" but not unattractive. That was only my opinion. The important thing was she was still unhappy.

Nearly every one of the forty or so plastic surgeons in the room congratulated the doctor on his result and said the woman should be happy with her result. "She's crazy," was one dismissive assessment.

The room murmured with agreement and self-satisfaction, whereupon I inserted myself into the impending maelstrom by stating rather matter-of-factly, "You all say she should be happy, but obviously she's not. It's interesting that a room full of white males is trying to tell an Asian woman how she should feel about her nose."

Well, you would have thought I had placed a black Swastika, a burning cross, and Mao's Little Red Book in the middle of the living room! They obviously thought they alone possessed the truth to the patient's own self. Perhaps I shouldn't have said "white" or maybe not "male," but one of the surgeons actually called my comments "racist." My subsequent, rather innocent, retort, made in jest, of course, was a suggestion to present photos of his Caucasian male face at a meeting in Shanghai and see how forty female Chinese surgeons would operate on his very own proboscis, or something to that effect. The room was immediate quieted with a few scattered snickers. Hopefully I said it with just enough humor to make my point since I consider the surgeon a good friend and colleague.

What we plastic surgeons think is not necessarily as important as what our patients think. In another example played out in a collection of articles, editorials, and commentary letters published in the official journal of our national society, a debate revolved around an age-old issue: What is the ideal size of breast implants for augmentation patients and how is that determined? Surgeons were commenting on the average size of implants each used in his practice. One respected surgeon stated that his average size was larger than another surgeon's because that was what his patients wanted, while the other criticized him for using implants that were too big and prone to more complications. Ignoring for the moment that the current method of measuring a patient for breast implants uses dimensions rather than volume, the concluding reply was the expected consumer warning, "caveat emptor" or "let the buyer beware." Let the buyer/patient have complete autonomy and responsibility for their choice; plastic surgeons should give them what they want even if they don't agree.

The second surgeon took the position that plastic surgeons should determine what is best for the patient since we have the advantage of knowledge and experience. Certainly, this fundamental difference in philosophy and practice has generated many lawsuits since each belief leads to different end results. One path might lead to an unhappy patient whose breasts are too small and the other to more complications and side effects. Both paths to larger breasts could, and usually do, statistically, lead to happy patients since the overall satisfaction rate is about ninety-five percent. But the fact that breast implants are fundamentally unnecessary, but desirable, means that even one dissatisfied patient is one too many.

* * *

So what is the truth? I believe the truth begins with the desire to search for the truth. That is, the goal of plastic surgery is not just in the doing of a procedure but it is the search for the reason patients are sitting in the well-appointed plastic surgeon's office decorated with the trophies of his education and accomplishments. If a patient doesn't know why he or she is sitting in the chair, then I can't be sure I will be able to help them. The truth can only be found if there is a conscious effort to find the truth. Like marriage counseling or psychotherapy, the effort to find answers is wasteful if one is not interested in finding the truth.

The patient and the doctor need to ask: What is the *goal* of this encounter? The goal cannot be assumed. There may be many goals with different relative priorities that are never voiced. If we are not tuned in to the search for that truth, we will never recognize it. We will never know if we are buying or selling the right item. Making a decision is not the same as understanding it. Making any decision is not identical to making the correct decision. The search for the truth leads us back to the patient. What is the play really about? Why is she sitting there? What does she fear? What does she desire? What is motivating her? How do I know I am going to make the patient happy if she herself doesn't know what will make her content and happy?

Simply being discontent with one's appearance is not a goal nor is it sufficient to make one a good candidate for plastic surgery. *Knowing what will make a person content is a mandatory first step.* If a salesman does not know what a customer is looking for, he cannot know if what he is selling is appropriate. Plastic surgeons cannot force their own ideas and approval on a patient, although we may try, like the room full of white, male surgeons discussing the nose of an Asian, female patient. Surprisingly, patients might even prefer this approach or be influenced by what is said from behind the mask of authoritative medical expertise. But buying and selling cosmetic surgery without knowing is a risky business, especially when you cannot easily return the purchase.

Many patients leave my office after a consultation deciding to forego or postpone surgery. Many accept themselves better and minimize the concern with their perceived imperfections. Other plastic surgeons and their surgical consultants may feel defeated when a patient rejects surgery but, while my income may suffer, I do not find this decision to be a disappointment. In fact, I often feel that I have done my job in making a person discover his or her own truth and feel better about him- or herself without even having to pick up a scalpel.

One attractive patient in her early forties sent me a cheerful thank-you note stating that after speaking with me, she acknowledged her fine wrinkles and looked at them as her badge of a life lived well. "I earned these wrinkles," she proclaimed to me in a heartfelt note. For her, cosmetic plastic surgery *was* unnecessary. She was able to say "no" and be happy. The result was found in her heart and between her ears.

The fact that plastic surgery is unnecessary makes the need to know what a patient desires imperative. From one discontent, there can be many possibilities. We can make a crooked nose with a droopy tip look like a thousand different noses. We can make a small breast into many different sizes and shapes. We can give an aging face an infinite number of rejuvenation choices, none of which is any more right or wrong, or good or bad, or normal or abnormal than the next; just look at all the variations in the world. If only we knew which variation to choose. **And the only way for us to know is for the patient to know.**

For every patient who decides that plastic surgery is not for her, there will be another who realizes that it is not only the loose skin of the eyelids that bothers her but also her jowls, and the fat under her neck and the hollow cheeks, and all the lines and folds. And maybe even the breasts and thighs. And her abdomen. And maybe even her ears. And that is okay. Some of my best and happiest patients are those who swore they wanted only one thing corrected. "I'll be fine; I'm not a plastic surgery junkie." Five years later, they have had multiple other concerns addressed to their satisfaction in a chart two inches thick.

Recently, a pleasant, very smart, sixty-five-year-old woman came in to see me. She was definitely in control of her life except as far as her appearance was concerned. She was assertive, opinionated, and self-assured. But she was also mildly diabetic and, despite a vigorous exercise routine, even with bad joints, knees, and hips, moderately obese. Her torso was burdened with extra skin and recalcitrant rolls of fat following a weight loss of nearly one hundred pounds. She initially just wanted her face to look the way it did two decades earlier. To her credit, she even brought in Photoshopped images to demonstrate exactly what she wanted. So I started with a scalp advancement to lower the forehead, facelift, mid-face lift, and neck lift. Elated by the results, she began to look for similar improvement elsewhere. After careful consultation in six office visits over half a year's period, I proceeded with a breast reduction and liposuction of her lateral chest fat rolls and upper abdomen. This was followed by serial liposuction of her abdomen and surgical excision of her lateral chest fat rolls, and six weeks later, completion of her staged abdominoplasty. Her recent surgeries to date were bilateral brachioplasties to contour her flapping arm tissues, and implants and a lift to give her fuller breasts. She is one of my happiest and most grateful patients.

* * *

As I discuss desires with the patient, her life will start to unfold. She begins to talk about her childhood, her successes, and her failures. She reveals her expectations of life and her fears of the future. She divulges uncertainties about employment or romance. She uncovers dissatisfaction with looking like her mother or becoming like her father. One young woman who had her surgery documented on a reality television show confessed to me, and the world, that she felt like an ugly duckling compared to her more attractive identical twin sister. After I did her surgery, including a rhinoplasty and breast augmentation, she began a career as a model.

A patient will commit to what bothers her and hopefully not commit to what does not. She will begin to make specific choices about specific features or specific body parts: a sharply defined nasal tip, fullness in the upper pole of the breast, a smooth jaw line, elimination of this wrinkle or that fold of tissue. A vision starts to take shape.

It is only by acknowledging that the plastic surgery she is about to have is unnecessary that the patient can reclaim the responsibility and the power for her decisions and give herself a fighting chance at finding her own truth. She needs to know the ramifications of her options, but only *she* can judge *which* option fulfills her honest desires.

One practical example is in breast enlargement. We all know patients want to be bigger. But I also want to know if she comes out bigger or smaller than expected, which would make her *more unhappy*; unhappiness is the complication to be avoided. The answer she is forced to give is another piece of her own truth. It is truly remarkable when asked this seemingly simple and innocent question how some patients can answer it with unwavering certainty and others struggle back and forth with their answer.

Once the patient's desire is made known, and that may be a daunting and arduous task worthy of more than a ten-minute consultation with a surgical consultant, then the ball is in my hands to determine how close I can get to that desire and what it will take to accomplish the task. But that is the easy part for me. Creating, designing, and envisioning a goal are difficult. Executing it is a practiced skill. Or as Albert Einstein prioritized it, imagination is often worth more than knowledge.

Forcing a patient to be an active participant is not the same as leaving the medical decision solely in her hands since I must critique and communicate the ramifications of any decision as I see them. Some desires are impossible to achieve, and some are dangerous to attempt. The decision-making process is *collaborative medicine* between the patient as a customer or client and the plastic surgeon as artist and technician. As in a healthy marriage, each must honestly communicate his or her thoughts and respect each other's opinion. Both marriage and plastic surgery can make life a lot more enjoyable and fulfilling. Both involve the search for one's own true self in the face of the question: What do I desire? Both are really unnecessary...but desirable.

CHAPTER 3:

INCISIVE BEGINNINGS

* * *

Before there is the patient, there is the surgeon. If this endeavor called cosmetic surgery is really collaboration, then how I formulate my responsibilities and my view of what I do will obviously affect what happens to my patient. So what has been my journey? Where did my approach to cosmetic plastic surgery come from? It certainly did not begin in Beverly Hills.

My father, Robert Hsun-Piao Yuan, was born in the Chinese seaport city of Ningbo in 1922. When he was a toddler, he lost his mother, a teacher, to scarlet fever. He and one of his seven sisters also contracted the infection but survived. His father remarried but died when he was five, leaving him and his half-brother, John, to be cared for by his stepmother, his minister grandfather, and his older sisters. He spent his summers of innocence catching crickets for playful cricket fights and cracking dried watermelon seeds for baking pastries. His memory of his early childhood was filled with happiness. He vividly remembered the fun and games with his schoolmates and, later in high school, with his numerous cousins and siblings. Yet even at an early age, he saw a purpose, a calling, to his life.

My father's maternal grandfather, the first Chinese consecrated bishop, infused my father with Christian ideology. This continued throughout his entire formal education from high school, college, and medical school at the prestigious missionary school, St. John's University in Shanghai, where one of his uncles eventually became the president. With remarkable observation and intuition, my father recognized that China had few neurosurgeons and set himself on a path to become one in order to help his countrymen. It is easy to follow a father's footstep or to aspire to what one sees in front of him. It is a different foresight to perceive and forge a path creating what is missing. That sounds more like what a plastic surgeon does.

Surviving the onslaught of the Japanese invasion during World War II, my father completed his college and medical school education as president of his class while his uncle endured the criticism by the Nationalist government that he had conspired with the puppet government to protect the university from the Japanese. At the same time, my mother, Grace I Chen, the pretty, outspoken and independent daughter of Bishop Robin Chen, who later became the presiding bishop of the Anglican Church in China, was completing her degree at Ginling Girl's College in Nanking. As a student leader who once represented China at an international youth conference in India in 1947 with Prime Minister Nehru in attendance, she was never lacking in boldness and confidence. Undoubtedly, the constant moving about to escape the Japanese insurgence, often with the whole congregation of her father's diocese in tow, did little to dampen her fiery spirit. More likely, that experience fueled it further. Like a whole generation of Chinese students following the end of the World War, both my father and mother would, independent of each other, seek to further their education in the United States. They would meet at the University of Pennsylvania Medical School, half a world away.

My mother was the only one of the three women in her class to obtain her medical degree; according to her, the other two succumbed to suicide and emotional breakdown. Three days after her graduation in Philadelphia in 1952, my father and mother married. By now, their homeland had been firmly sealed from them by the Communist takeover in 1949. At the time, my mother's father, Bishop Chen, was helping to organize the state-sanctioned Church of China under the Mao-led Communist rule, enduring heavy criticism from Western religious leaders. This activity earned him the obviously disdainful moniker "the Red Bishop."

My father moved his new bride to Boston to join the neurosurgical staff at the Tufts-New England Medical Center. My mother began a short-lived clinical stint in pediatrics, and, having given birth to my two sisters and me, abandoned clinical medicine to do laboratory research in the field of tissue culture at Harvard and MIT. Now with two doctors in the family in the culturally and educationally rich, sports-obsessed city of Boston, Massachusetts, my path in life as their only son seemed obvious.

* * *

My earliest recollection of childhood was as a toddler at the Wollaston Lutheran School, solving math problems while sitting alone at a desk facing the wall in a large room full of more playful kindergartners. I guess that must have impressed upon me the value of higher cerebral function while suggesting that there was something different about me. I would go on to skip first grade and become the second grade teacher's pet, incurring immense embarrassment on one occasion while passing out blank sheets of writing paper to the other students who were sitting dutifully in their rows of wooden desks awaiting instructions for our spelling test. On this tragic day I had miscounted, a cardinal sin as the infallible teacher's pet; the second row was short one sheet of paper. It seems so trivial in retrospect but it felt monumental at the time. Being wrong was not a fun thing, especially in front of people who relied on, and trusted, me.

* * *

My days of youth were blessed. I played all kinds of sports (baseball, football, tennis, basketball, squash, ping pong) and learned the violin (giving recitals, performing with a youth symphony orchestra, even being handpicked by the great conductor Leopold Stokowski to join an international youth orchestra at a festival in Switzerland). I matriculated to Harvard and skipped my freshman year by passing three advanced placement examinations, including one in English, my least favorite subject, math, my easiest subject, and physics, my most challenging class in high school. Despite carrying as many as six full courses per semester, determined as I was to cram as much knowledge and experience as I could in three years of college, I remained diverse in my interests, choosing to avoid the common pre-med pathway of top-heavy science subjects. As such, I had the opportunity to study music and drama, economics, the history of science, Chinese language, Eastern philosophy, and the psychology of art, as well as the requisite organic chemistry and quantum mechanics. I graduated with honors at the tender age of nineteen. Although much of what I learned I'd forgotten, what I realized was that life is multidimensional and science is more art than science. Healthy skepticism leads to comfort in contrarian thinking, and narrow-mindedness is the enemy of truth.

The struggles of survival at Harvard, where everyone was someone and the university seemed to be at the center of the universe, forced me to find the strengths in myself. It required a constant effort to not drown in the surrounding sea of excellence. Along the way, I discovered the insecurities that I, like all humans, possessed, and as such, became privy to the individuality and uniqueness in every human being. That notion would stay with me throughout my plastic surgery training.

At the same time, my diverse interests and studies led me to the constant need to find the interrelatedness of human endeavor. There is commonality in playing the violin and in serving a tennis ball. The economics of supply and demand are applicable to the to and fro of interpersonal relationships. The emotions of a Puccini opera on stage are as intense as the emotions of surgical drama in the operating room. The art of the real estate deal is not unlike the matching of a plastic surgical procedure to a patient's aesthetic desires or reconstructive needs. My adventure in plastic surgery was about to begin.

* * *

As a third-year student at Harvard Medical School, I took a two-week elective rotation in plastic surgery at the Peter Bent Brigham Hospital, one of the premier Harvard-affiliated hospitals in the Boston area. Despite being the son of doctors, I was as ignorant about this specialty as one could be. I didn't even know why they called it "plastic" surgery. Cosmetic surgery was unheard-of in our brain surgeon's household, even though I had accompanied my father into his operating room numerous times before I was even a teenager.

Under the expansive and nurturing mind of my mentors, including future Nobel laureate Dr. Joseph Murray, subsequently named as one of the ten greatest plastic surgeons of the twentieth century by our professional society, I was mainly exposed to what was considered reconstructive: burn reconstruction, wound care, correction of congenital deformities. In each problem, I could see that individualized analysis and customized planning was necessary to attain the functional goal. You could not apply the exact same formula to each surgical problem. Each case was a new creative endeavor with its own nuances. One had to apply knowledge and imagination to each and every problem. Sometimes the solution seemed so obvious it was compelling to look for a different and better way. Sometimes there were too many choices. Sometimes there were no solutions and we had to invent one.

Being a classically trained violinist, I sensed it was not unlike playing great music: never the same, never taken for granted, never merely repetitive, always open to new interpretation—no cookie-cutter music, no cookie-cutter surgery, but also staying true to a surgical score. A lot of planning and thinking went into each case.

I once read that my childhood musical hero, Jascha Heifetz, the greatest violinist of the twentieth century, was appalled to discover, upon reviewing the sheet music of Chausson's *Poeme* (a favorite piece that I played at my last public recital back in medical school), that he had been performing the piece incorrectly for years. He took for granted that what he was playing was correct. It was not. The challenge is to not only play it correctly but to also play it uniquely and vice versa. Just like cosmetic surgery.

While I was training in general surgery as a prerequisite to further plastic surgical training, the emphasis in my experience continued to be on reconstructive cases: decubitus care, trauma, hand surgery, cancer surgery. Cosmetic surgery was seen as the coveted dessert anticipated as a just reward for tackling the substantial, and often less appetizing, main course. You put in your dues taking care of trauma and cancer patients so you could eventually bask in the delicious, sweet glamour of aesthetic surgery.

I had the opportunity to see premier surgeons in Los Angeles perform breast augmentations, facelifts, and rhinoplasty procedures. But many surgeons, touting their own adopted techniques or personal aesthetic senses, seemed to be offering up procedures to patients as definitive items, like clothes off the rack or pies from the dessert cart. Even as surgeons debated the merits of this or that procedure, interaction between the surgeon and patients was minimal. Patients basically came in for whatever the surgeon could offer them, whatever he favored for whatever reason. I was surprised how motivated, but passive, patients were in altering their bodies. It was like closing their eyes and trusting their hairdresser with the latest style. Even with the biggest celebrities, or especially with them, a lot of magical hand waving seemed to suffice for real consultations. Very few patients asked important, probing questions.

Then, having burnt out in medicine, presumably because I had completed two Harvard degrees by age twenty-three and because general surgical training with its long hours was so tedious, repetitive, and non-creative (we learned by "practicing" procedures, perhaps reliving why kids, my son included, hate practicing piano), I did the unthinkable. I did what no resident in a competitive, highly desirable, and prestigious surgical residency would ever think of doing. I went against the conventional advice of my father, my professors, and my fellow residents. I quit medicine.

I spent two years exercising another side of my body and brain playing music, writing screenplays, and teaching tennis. I traveled to China in the nascent days of its Western-style free enterprise experiment of the early 1980s, foretelling of the capitalist boom of China today. This economic "opening up" of China clashed with the palpable paranoia of the intellectuals and artists who feared a repeat of the Cultural Revolution, where a call for free expression brought on severe repression. You could literally feel the hunger for knowledge and freedom. People practiced their rudimentary English on one another in dimly lit parks and crowded boulevards. Free-market businesses sprung up in narrow, poorly lit alleys. They seemed inspired by what the unknown future held, foretelling the immense economic expansion in China in the decades to come.

Little did I know that I was nurturing my mind and soul for a more comprehensive approach to medicine: more humanistic, more creative, more thoughtful, more philosophical, more truthful *to myself.* Having stepped off the predetermined, regimented route of medical training for the first time since graduating college, I was primed for what Harvard was initially all about: veritas, the search for truth—not what is necessary, but what is desired. It was not so much about what I was doing in surgery or how I was doing it but *why* I was doing it. I didn't want to practice surgery by rote. Of course, at the time, the concept hadn't gelled so concretely, but it was there, lurking in the depths of my heart and mind, waiting to torture and inspire me for the next twenty years of my life. I felt rejuvenated and returned to medicine.

* * *

My formal plastic surgery training in Miami came under the creative genius of D. Ralph Millard, Jr., a giant contributor to the field of plastic surgery, which also earned him a rightful place as yet another of our ten greatest plastic surgeons of the twentieth century. Through exposure to his erudite, witty, creative, and very accessible writing expounding on his principles of plastic surgery, and his tying these to principles of human endeavors in war, football, boxing, and business, I came to believe that the practice of plastic surgery was something more than just a way to earn a living. His book, *Principlization of Plastic Surgery,* delineating his thirty-three principles, was a real eye-opener for me. I began to look for my own overriding philosophy to connect the dots of life and work.

I felt a need to reconcile my life as a doctor with life in general, to see the universal threads of truth running through both, perhaps like a religion, alluding back to the time-honored commitment of medicine as a calling. Even though I might not have been literally "saving lives" like my father did before me, my vocation as a plastic surgeon needed to be more than just "providing a service" or "purveying a product." My father's admonition to me, "You *must* have a purpose" rang constant in my mind. I also knew my patients would be better served if I was armed with a philosophical vision, with something more than a convenient truth. It is arrogant to think that a plastic surgeon can be a god—a savior and creator—although we are often accused of that notion. But we do want to have a positive impact on a patient's life.

* * *

"Doc, can you fix my nose?" she asked.
What do you mean by fix*?* I thought.

My initial decade in private practice in Los Angeles was primarily based in hospital settings, performing breast reconstructions, wound care and cancer surgery, lower extremity reconstruction with all types of pedicle or free flaps, cleft lip and palate reconstruction, facial fracture repair and craniofacial reconstruction, and even a bit of burn care. It was like reliving my residency but as a private doctor. In some ways, it was heaven. I felt needed, appreciated, and purposeful.

I did "fix" things. I made people whole. I took the cruel jokes nature played on a baby born with a cleft lip and made it so he could laugh proudly at that joke a decade later. I helped mend the body of a rock-and-roll singer whose leg was torn asunder by a chance meeting between his motorcycle and a car running a red light, and made it possible for that mangled leg to support his body dancing on a spotlighted stage. I lifted the spirit of a young executive, a doctor's daughter, whose breasts were both taken by cancer and gave her a left breast of self-confidence and a right breast of determination such that she was able to continue her productive life advocating for animals in need. The goals, priorities, and methods were clear. Doctors trusted me; I have taken on close to two hundred doctors and their family members as patients over the years. But *fixing* a nose? That was an entirely different challenge. *What's* wrong *with your nose?* I would think.

As I began to see more patients requesting cosmetic procedures, it was obvious that everyone, insurance companies, referring physicians, patients, and society in general, viewed cosmetic patients and cosmetic cases quite differently than reconstruction patients and reconstruction cases. There seemed to be a true dichotomy with a demilitarized gray zone of ambiguity between the two. In private practice, financial considerations set these two subspecialties apart; insurance might pay for reconstructive cases but never for cosmetic cases. *Medical necessity* was an industry catchphrase used to categorize each case. Reconstructive cases required medically necessary restoration of normal anatomy and function while cosmetic surgery provided no obvious medical, only merely psycho-emotional, benefit. Reconstructive cases were performed out of need within the all-powerful insurance system. Cosmetic cases were performed on demand outside the system. Reconstructive cases were a necessity. Cosmetic cases were a desire.

But insurance definitions are controlled by external financial and political considerations, not intrinsic truisms. Sometimes an insurance company would cover something you wouldn't think they would cover and not cover things you would swear should be covered. The solutions and decision-making process in reconstructive cases were challenging at times but made easier by the presence of various constraints: health of the patient, adequacy of blood supply, availability of autogenous tissue, age of the patient, the magnitude of what was to be gained in the event of a successful outcome. The goals were usually quite clear and the restrictions numerous. With cosmetic surgery, goals were often fuzzy and open-ended and what was to be gained seemed elusive at times. Yet what could be lost was monumental. I didn't realize this during training since, as residents, we just learned "how to do" and not always "why." We were focused on increasing the numbers of facelifts, rhinoplasties, and breast augmentations under our belts. The subdivisions of the specialty really did feel different then. Yet I felt uncomfortable with this dichotomy that seemed so artificial in many ways.

Are cosmetic surgery/cosmetic surgeons and reconstructive surgery/reconstructive surgeons so mutually exclusive of each other, as some patients believe? I think not because most cosmetic surgeons are products of reconstructive surgery education and cosmetic procedures are often adaptations of reconstructive techniques. Aren't they equal and interrelated parts of the whole field of plastic surgery? Can surgeons rationalize surgery in reconstructive cases based on proven physiology and strict statistical analysis and then be whimsical in cosmetic ones? Decision-making in cosmetic surgery *had* to be rationalized by something just as it was in reconstructive surgery. Can you believe in God while attending church but then become an atheist at a baseball game?

Again, there was the search for an all-purpose truth; one truth is that we are all structurally no more or less than just a composite of anatomy: bone, cartilage, blood vessels, nerves, lymphatics, fat, skin, etc. That's it. It doesn't matter if you are a reconstructive patient or a cosmetic patient. How can we approach cosmetic surgery and reconstructive surgery so differently, but still possess a commonality in anatomy and techniques? And what is the rationalization for cosmetic procedures: what the patient wants, what a surgeon is capable of, what a surgeon likes, or what is in vogue? Good doctors need to rationally justify their actions, *every* action, especially in surgery that one might consider to be unnecessary.

As I performed more cosmetic surgery, it became clear to me that I needed a philosophy or a belief system to answer the practical and theoretical questions patients posed when seeking cosmetic surgery: When do I need surgery? How long will the results of this procedure last? Is this new procedure better than the old? What will make me look good? Are *you* any good? What do you think? Will this operation be worth it? Will I look natural? All these routine questions with seemingly routine answers were so difficult to answer.

I wondered if I was missing something in my training that might have failed me in my ability to perform

cosmetic surgery but that I seemed to possess effort-
lessly in reconstructive cases. Would I really have to
completely re-educate and re-invent myself to deal
with cosmetic patients? I knew that giving a patient
a healthy, functional leg after suffering a compound,
comminuted fracture with soft tissue loss would
improve his life, as would creating a normal-appear-
ing lip from a cleft deformity, but would smoothing
the wrinkles on someone's neck or reducing the bags
under her eyes do the same? I felt more nervous operating on cosmetic, rather than reconstructive, patients.
I knew I had to find truth in order to answer patients
honestly and with conviction.

At times, doctors seemed to provide inadequate
answers to patients (perhaps because it was conventional wisdom, politically correct, or financially motivated) and I found myself very skeptical of these
answers. How did a doctor know a patient would look
"fabulous"? Why did he think he could "fix" a patient's
nose that wasn't "broken" or make a woman feel more
beautiful when she couldn't even see her own face
except in mirrors and photographs? How could he
know her facelift would last seven years when he didn't
know what she would look like in seven years *without*
the facelift? Why should a patient assume her breast
lift would look like all the other breast lifts in his brag
book, and if it didn't, why was he showing pictures to
her in the first place? How could a surgeon bring a
patient to a happy destination when the patient didn't
know where she wanted to go? I knew I wasn't stupid,
so if I found the answers inadequate, then so might
patients. The answer was in part to look at cosmetic
surgery more as art and less as science. Ask whether

Van Gogh's *Portrait of Dr. Gachet* is worth eighty-two and a half million dollars, and see what answers you get.

Cosmetic surgery was more challenging a field than I had imagined. Given my very practical Episcopalian and high-minded Harvard education, the constant nagging I felt to put it all into perspective spurred me on to find more meaningful answers to these common questions. Being in Beverly Hills seems like an obvious first choice for the practice of cosmetic surgery, but has also proven to be the perfect setting for feeling like a fish out of water. Here is where I formulated my *philosophy* of cosmetic surgery, ironically something very few patients, if any, ever think about.

CHAPTER 4:

THE FIFTH DIMENSION

"The problem with men and women is that they want different things: men want women and women want men."
—Attributed to W.C. Fields

* * *

Since entering plastic surgery, I've searched for some *structure* to the freethinking and creative spirit that is attractive and necessary in this field. To some extent, this search for *order* seems like a contradiction that is bound to disappoint, frustrate, and destroy that same creativity. Yet as Rudolf Arnheim, my professor of the psychology of art at Harvard, said, "Order is a necessary condition for anything the human mind is to understand."[1] On the other hand, with my musical education, I knew that one had to extend oneself beyond the regimented order found in black notes written on musical staffs and, only then, discover the *meaning* to those notes. As Arnold Steinhardt, the violinist of the famed Guarneri Quartet, in his autobiography, *Violin Dreams*, quoting the great cellist Pablo Casals, writes, this demands *"freedom with order."* How

1 Arnheim, R., Entropy and Art, (1971) University of California Press, Berkeley

can you be loyal to artistic creativity and freedom but also be held accountable to, and perhaps constrained by, some higher ideal besides mere anatomical normalcy? And how can you do this while simultaneously giving patients what *they* want?

I can imagine God thinking about how to create human beings. "How do I give a person two eyes, two ears, a nose, a mouth, four limbs, a head, and a body without creating out of mere randomness like some distorted Picasso portrait, and yet not produce a world of clones?" Well, He or She obviously figured it out: ordered similarity with infinite variation.

As I learned the mechanics of plastic surgery, I argued against the dogmatic, by rote, or repetitive approach to cosmetic surgery that led me away from the other surgical specialties in the first place. I am uncomfortable with the standard recipes that are called for in rhinoplasties, facelifts, and breast reductions. Despite sounding like an oxymoron, *structured creativity* is something I always felt must exist and, even more importantly, is essential if I truly believe in what I do in my profession. It goes to the very core of what it means to be a plastic surgeon: why I do what I do, and what I want out of my "job." The answer justifies my existence and value. Without it, I end up only doing what others tell or teach me to do—a mere technician—or, alternatively, I can arrogantly, and justifiably, do anything I want without accountability because I am "The Doctor." As an artist, it is either like painting by numbers and thus reproducing art mechanically by some formula or pattern versus throwing paint against a wall and calling it art for no good reason except that it might be expressive. How can I favorably compare plastic surgery, if it is considered an artistic endeavor, to any other artistic field, whether it is music, painting, filmmaking, literature, or even cartoons? What can move plastic surgery above technical exercises, repetitive pigeonholing, or unconstrained chaos even as medicine as a whole gravitates towards uniformly prescribed protocols, outcome testing, and reproducible results? Is my search simply part of the universal pursuit for *truth* and *purpose* in one's work or is it a misguided exercise in futility? The fact that our world has infinite variation, but also definite order, is encouraging.

Part of the problem with my search is that the *measure of success* has to do with the *goal* of surgery. Outcome results have no meaning without agreement on the *value* of each outcome one measures. Ask parents how they define being successful at parenting or how they judge the success of their children and it will be clear that each person's value system is different. Ask financial analysts what is the most important indicator of a company's success and a grab bag of data will spew forth.

With most surgical procedures, the goal is quite clear and limited. In appendectomies, it is to remove the appendix. In oncological colon resection, it is to remove the tumor. In orthopedics, it is to mend the bones. Of course, it is, in reality, much more complicated since risks and side effects need to be taken into account, but how one measures success and, more especially, why one does surgery at all is narrowly defined. Much of the time, the goal of the surgeon and the goal of the patient are aligned. Both want the inflamed appendix out, the cancer in the colon gone, and the broken bones healed. One can report that surgery was or was not a success based on narrow parameters. In reconstructive plastic surgery where anatomy is abnormal from trauma, congenital development, or surgical treatment, the goal is generally presumed to be to *restore normal form and function.* The closer the final form resembles normal anatomy with normal function, the more successful the surgery.

All surgeons prefer the definitiveness and concreteness of their tasks. That's why we are not internists or psychiatrists. We like to see evidence of the problem, design specific surgical maneuvers and manipulations, and visually witness the obvious benefits of our work. The black box of medicinal treatment makes many surgeons uncomfortable, whereby some abstract, intangible symptom like nausea, or bloating, or the worst symptom of all, pain, is affected by some pill that disappears into the mouth or is buried into the muscles by a needle and syringe and somehow circulates around the body unseen, hopefully influencing these symptoms without damaging something else. Medicines to surgeons are like secret and mystical ninjas deployed in the dark of night to accomplish some impossible task. Even in the use of topical and oral agents commonly seen in so-called anti-aging treatment that cosmetic plastic surgeons have embraced, the visual improvements are often slow, gradual, qualitative, and even unpredictable. It's all rather magical and mysterious. If one throws in the placebo effect, it can turn a well-trained surgeon into a skeptic and cynic.

Plastic surgeons, in particular, are very visual. If we can't see it, we can't fix it (although some critics accuse us of doing exactly that). If we can't photograph it, we can't judge it. How we assess our work, in general, relates to how it looks; not many blind people get cosmetic surgery. Yet in my educational travels through the world of cosmetic patients, I am impressed by how often the assessments by patients are not in agreement with the assessments by their surgeons and sometimes even less so with others around them.

The standard for success in each patient seems elusive and possibly contradictory. I often squirm when I hear patients gush how happy they are with a result that I would rate mediocre. Some results are even dangerous, like a slender and pointed nasal tip on an Asian patient produced by a silicone implant that has all likelihood of eroding through the nose in the future. At the same time, I sweat in confusion (oh, for the grace of God go I) when I hear other patients complain bitterly about a result of which any surgeon would be proud. I often hear patients criticize a surgeon for not listening to them or accuse a doctor with "Look what that he did to me!" Even more disturbing are the disagreements some spouses or partners have that expose the core of their relationship, whether fragile or rock-solid, and that reveal the deep effect cosmetic surgery has on patients, deeper than what is obviously visualized.

How can I unleash surgical creativity while allaying my fears of going against the traditional ethical code in medicine of "Primum non nocere" or "First, do no harm"? How can one *not* possibly do harm when operating on perfectly *normal* people? Tales of doctors being charged with battery on disgruntled patients make the need for a rational, practical, yet philosophical paradigm even more compelling. I have to find that overriding construct that guides my hand in surgery. I have to understand the *goal* of cosmetic surgery better.

As with any surgical field, I have to go to its begin-nings; in the beginning, with surgery, "it's all about the anatomy, stupid!" (Not you, the reader, "stupid," but we, the surgeons, "stupid.") *All surgery relates to human anatomy.* Surgeons do not work on molecules, ideations, or feelings. We cannot will an effect. Wishful thinking will not change the way we are built. We work on the anatomy. We cannot possibly change human structure without analyzing that structure. Cosmetic plastic surgery is no different and is simply the manip-ulation of anatomy to create a certain aesthetic and visual result. That is basically all it is: *applied anatomy.* Before anyone asks what will make them younger, or better, or more attractive, or how much something costs, or if liposuction, contour threads, implants, or lasers work or not, you have to start with the anatomy.

Humans are all constructed out of the same mate-rial. We are just arranged differently. We all have a skeletal structure of bones and cartilage. We have soft tissue components of fat, nerves, blood vessels, and muscle. We have a covering of dermis, skin and its pig-mentation and appendages like hair, sweat glands, oil glands, etc. As long as we have the right combination, amount, and form of these anatomical components, we can theoretically build any human body. Artists, both computer-based and physical medium-based, employ this anatomical basis of the human form.

One obvious, often overlooked, aspect to this con-cept is that human anatomy is three-dimensional. Computer-generated images are two-dimensional rep-resentations of this three-dimensional form; so, too, are photographs and drawings that are ubiquitous in medical education and in the mass media to which patients so readily refer. The three-dimensionality of human anatomy is precisely why cadaver dissection in human anatomy labs is so critical, most often beginning the very first year of medical school. It is why many new techniques in surgery require dissection and practice on human subjects (dead or alive) when initially being developed or subsequently taught. We cannot judge or make recommendations on noses or faces or breasts by scrutinizing two-dimensional photographs, especially on one view alone. Usually, we rely on our visual perception and cortical, as well as limbic, functions to convert a two-dimensional representation into a three-dimensional understanding and visualization. Some people/patients are good at this and some have very little aptitude. This ability of conceptualizing spatial relationships is mainly a right-brain function, leading to the observation that many plastic surgeons, including me, are left-handed.

The fact that the human body is a three-dimensional object requires us, specifically as plastic surgeons, to define each and every patient in three-dimensional anatomic terms. That is, when I look at a female patient, I initially see her in objective everyday terms, such as a blond or brunette Caucasian, or an elderly Chinese woman with facial wrinkles, or a shapely girl with a pooching abdomen and flat chest, or a mother, or your Aunt Tilly. I just see the objective form and shape without placing any *value* judgment on what I see. I am not dissecting the individual's anatomy. That will come later when I must acknowledge that despite the similarities of every human being, we are all anatomically different. Even identical twins have minute differences in their anatomy.

Putting on my surgeon's cap and observing further, I then must define the patient's features in exacting anatomical terms. This is where the examination comes in. From this examination and knowledge of human anatomy, a three-dimensional construct of the patient is produced that allows me to understand why the patient looks the way she does, why she is unique, and what anatomical features make her the individual she is (i.e., why Aunt Tilly looks like Aunt Tilly). Sometimes I need a simple laying-on of hands or a studious visual survey with a keen, trained eye. Sometimes I need a radiographic image to determine this. Often I take measurements, particularly of breasts, and I always take multi-view photographs. I can then make assessments based solely on three-dimensional, anatomical features without emotional interpretation.

Now I see a teenage girl with a hump on the nasal bridge caused by projections of nasal bone, septal cartilage, and thick dermis, or a middle-aged woman with an obtuse angle to the chin and neck caused by a recessive mandible, lax skin, and a thick layer of fat over her loose platysmal muscle, or an elderly gentleman who has folds or wrinkles of the face caused by atrophic skin with a paucity of fat hanging on hypoplastic malar bones. The anatomy starts to take on definition, meaning, and emotional significance. It is a distinctly unique way of looking at a human being that is different than a layperson's view. I begin to visually dissect the person's anatomy sort of like the voyeur who undresses his subjects with his eyes.

Anthropometric and cephalometric measurements can help define or categorize three-dimensional human form. While these mathematically and sociologically based data cannot define beauty or attractiveness (although researchers have attempted to), they may be able to help us gauge the relative normalcy of a person's anatomy and can verify or guide a surgical game plan to change the anatomy. For example, if one suspects that a patient might benefit from a chin advancement or implant, measuring the position of the bony chin point (menton) and soft tissue projection of the chin (pogonion) and slope of her mandible relative to her lips, her nasal spine (subnasale), her nasal tip, her nasal root (glabella), something called Frankfort's horizontal or Frankfort's plane, and Rickett's E line may support or refute this assessment. But even this meticulously detailed and complex analysis won't tell us if and how any chin augmentation should be performed. The same can be said for the myriad of measurements I take in analyzing breasts. At this stage, I am more like an engineer than an architect.

Rarely should plastic surgeons operate on pure, raw, numerical data. Besides ignoring the fact that there are wide variations in beauty and attractiveness, fitting all patients into a mathematical model produces individuals that all look similar. How science fiction-like! But that is precisely why patients start to look alike...until they all arrive at the "done" look, unrecognizable as unique individuals.

Even in breast augmentation, seemingly one of the simplest operations in plastic surgery, anatomical nuances, some not even apparent to trained surgeons, will produce significant effects on results. Conceptually, breast augmentation is fairly basic, mindless, and perhaps crude; surgeons stick something foreign under the breast that increases volume. The history of breast enlargement has seen surgeons use paraffin, ivory, gutta-percha, ox-based cartilage, liquid silicone, polyvinyl, polyether, and polyurethane materials. Luckily we have evolved from some of these disastrous implants to prostheses that are quite well tolerated. However, even in today's rather well-developed (pardon the pun) techniques, without detailed microscopic analysis of anatomy, minute elements like asymmetrical curvature of the rib cage, size and potential projection of the nipple and subareolar breast tissue, relative position of the breasts to the clavicle and width of the chest, presence of scoliosis or postural habits, differences in soft tissue distribution of each breast, and relative thickness of the chest wall muscles may go undetected and can influence the final result.

Now having an idea of the patient's specific anatomy and having satisfied the first three dimensions of the problem, the fourth dimension of time can be factored in. The fourth dimension of time comes into play because the human body is not a static object. The anatomy is constantly moving and changing. Sometimes it is the moment to moment changes, as occurs with muscular activity, producing dynamic facial wrinkles (the ones that Botox targets), or posture, producing unsightly skin folds or fat bulges (as when one bends the neck or sits down), or the changes that relate to soft tissue pliability or elasticity, which is basically the ability to change shape over a momentary period of time. Sometimes it is the longer-interval changes brought on by fluid intake, weight fluctuations, pregnancy, the aging process, and gravity.

Even hard structures like bone can change over one's lifetime. We know that bone remodels naturally, with some areas in the face being osteoclastic (resorptive) and some being osteoblastic (additive). Bone is influenced by pressure of overlying implants as in the face, chin, and breast, by the presence and use of teeth, as in the maxilla and mandible, by trauma, and by over- or under-use of muscles.

Sometimes the temporal changes in the anatomy are the reasons the patient is sitting in my office: She used to look a certain way and now, X years later, she looks different. It may not even be the specific features but the *changes* of the features that have occurred over the years that bother the patient. *The only constant that doesn't change is change itself.*

The full analysis of a patient's anatomy must take these temporal changes into consideration. As a result, pictures revealing the temporal changes are immensely helpful and I always request photos from a patient's past to see *what* those changes are in order to understand *how* those changes occurred. Looking at a photograph taken at one moment in time is like trying to understand a movie looking at just one frame. You need to see a sequence over time to know if the person is walking forwards or backwards and to know how fast they are walking and with what demeanor. Personal, face-to-face, hands-on examination is imperative in this analysis. A breast made out of fat and glandular tissue will move and feel quite different than that same breast made of clay or a hardened breast implant. A photograph will not suffice. A face at rest will look different and show different features when animating. Bilateral facial paralysis as in Mobius syndrome will not show up in a static photograph. A torso will produce a different shape when the abdominal muscles are contracting or when the posture is changed. That is why my examination of a patient seeking to improve her abdominal contour always includes asking her to stand naturally, to stand straight, to flex at the waist, and to contract the abdominal muscles with and without inhaling. I need to assess these dynamic qualities.

Live examination is critical in analyzing a patient. Photographic representations of patients can be influenced by lighting, position, and muscle activity. For example, brows can be made to look higher or lower by the position of the camera and whether the patient is looking up or straight ahead. The degree to which a patient's abdomen protrudes may be dependent on his abdominal muscle tone and posture. One can only distinguish banding in the neck caused by loose skin versus hyperactive platysmal muscle by observing the patient contracting his neck muscles.

Modern photographic techniques allow time-lapsed morphing to reveal both subtle and dramatic temporal effects of aging. By overlaying photographs taken over time of specific body regions, surgeons can observe a person's anatomic life as if in a movie. This can provide invaluable clues as to how and why the patient appears more aged. With the help of this technology, downward drooping of facial soft tissue has proved to be less important in aging than once thought. Rather, it may be the deflationary effect of fat atrophy that influences facial aging more and gives rise to the popularity of injectable fillers to restore volume to the face.

The other aspect to the fourth dimension is to relate the expected, and unexpected, changes that surgery is designed to produce. It can be used to guide the patient through the post-operative period, when anatomical changes due to the many phases of swelling, bruising, and scarring may be temporary. A lot of handholding and gentle admonishment to avoid looking at the operative site immediately after surgery can save a patient's emotional sense of well-being. I often tell patients that examining a result too soon is like a chef constantly peeking in the oven and tasting a turkey before it is cooked. It will only frustrate and mislead them. The temporary changes of post-operation need to abate before true assessment of a surgical result can take place. Even then, we know that the human body is constantly changing through time. What a person looks like today may not be what he looks like in six months and it won't be what he looks like in a decade. Thus, judgment pre- and post-surgery will be dependent on the time interval; *nothing is forever.*

Anyone going through pregnancy, childbirth, breast-feeding, severe weight changes, intensive physical training, extreme emotional stress, or puberty knows how quickly and drastically a human body and its various parts can change. Aging can be graceful but also quite abrupt. Post-operative alterations produce nearly instantaneous, and persistently varying, changes.

For example, in rhinoplasty, we try to produce fixed, hard tissue structures by reducing, moving, adding, suturing, or grafting bone and cartilage, yet the overlying soft tissues, because of their intricately related and minutely sensitive nature, can obscure the true post-operative results for months. Bruising, swelling, scarring, contraction, and softening all take effect to varying degrees at overlapping times. Carried to its logical extreme, the nose a twenty-year-old patient possesses a year after surgery will probably not be the nose he or she places bifocal glasses on at age sixty. These changes, however gradual and imperceptible, still occur whether or not we wish to acknowledge them.

A practical, yet also rhetorical, question frequently posed to plastic surgeons is, "When am I healed?" It is when the temporal changes related to surgery have subsided to the point of being imperceptible. That can be three weeks or one year. It isn't a distinct moment in time.

Now that the four dimensions of human physical appearance and anatomy are defined and understood, some *judgment* must be rendered. We begin to assign *emotional value* to that anatomy. Instead of seeing Aunt Tilly, we might see an Aunt Tilly who is looking older and more tired than before. Instead of seeing a middle-aged, white-haired woman, we might see an out-of-shape woman who seems depressed. Instead of seeing a young male with a square jaw and prominent cheeks, we might see a handsome hunk of a chiseled-featured man with a sexy demeanor or, similarly, when we see a woman with almond eyes, high cheekbones, and an hourglass figure, we might see a sensuous, attractive woman with elegance and class. We determine if a certain feature is good or bad; is there too much or not enough of something? Is it desirable or undesirable? Is it attractive or not? Here, a myriad of influences will produce this *judgment* from cultural teachings, religious points of view, fashion trends, familial traits, pop culture icons, childhood experiences, parental values, and individual aesthetic senses.

Patients need to form *psycho-emotional* opinions of their anatomical features. But beyond this, they must be able to communicate this opinion to plastic surgeons and the surgeon must be able to see the patient through the patient's eyes. It is the "Aha!" moment when the two have a *meeting of the minds* that the surgical work can then begin. The four dimensions of human existence are only analytical and retrospective. They can only describe what exists. They only describe what we see. They do not assign emotional value, require opinions, or guide creativity. They do not describe what we have yet to feel. They do not tell me what I should do or not do surgically.

The **fifth dimension refers to the psycho-emotional feelings about, and assessment of, a person's four-dimensional anatomy.** The goal and expectation is a mutual understanding and acceptance between a patient and the plastic surgeon. The fifth dimension is precisely the emotional motivation behind the reason patients are in my office to begin with. It will be the justification for entering the operating room. It will be the roadmap leading me in my surgical manipulation, and it will be the final determinant of the patient's happiness. **The fifth dimension is quite simply the embodiment of *plastic surgery as art*.** As Paul Eluard, the French poet, noted, "To see is to understand." That is the first step. But what you see will not be static. As Picasso put it, "A picture...changes as one's thoughts change... When it is finished, it still goes on changing, according to the state of mind of whoever is looking at it...a picture lives only through the person who is looking at it." For me, both that picture and that person are one and the same.

The fifth dimension is the reason there can be two diverse and diametrically opposed opinions of the same painting, piece of music, movie, or even human being. It speaks to the individuality of each patient and the need to not let prejudice, pre-judgment, or assumptions color the patient's and plastic surgeon's goal of doing what is appropriate. How many times have patients had doctors assume they wanted cheek implants when they really just wanted their nose changed, or upgrade their breasts to a C-cup when they only wanted a B-cup, or presume they would like their thighs suctioned when all they desired was a slightly flatter abdomen following childbirth? The fifth dimension also obviously argues against standard, by-rote approaches to cosmetic problems. While the fifth dimension is related to and requires the other four dimensions, it is necessarily independent of them, just as all mathematical dimensions are independent of each other. As I explain to patients, a set of twins with exactly the same anatomy may end up with different surgical solutions because what they each think is attractive may be different. In fact, they may be affected psycho-emotionally in completely opposite ways by their identical features.

The fifth dimension is also why generalizations in cosmetic surgery are not helpful. What a "typical" Asian nose is like is not very helpful to an individual Chinese patient. What ninety-nine other patients did for their breast augmentation is not helpful to the one patient now sitting in front of me. The patient's girlfriend's or spouse's opinion is only relevant to me as it influences the patient's own opinion.

There are practical issues to this rather philosophical constraint, as one can see. Intrinsic to this concept of the fifth dimension is the need for knowing one's patient and a patient knowing one's plastic surgeon. *Communication is essential.* When a nurse or salesperson acts as the primary go-between, as is the case in many plastic surgeons' offices, information is often misrepresented, even if unintentional. Some *mis*directed information could be by design since the function of the go-between may be to "close" the financial deal.

This presents another opportunity for a margin of error. A patient's concern may be minimized because it hinders the closing of the deal. It is not uncommon for patients who are unhappy about their surgery to complain that they never talked to the surgeon and had things translated or explained mainly by someone other than the surgeon. They might have implicitly trusted the surgeon to do "what was right" without really knowing or agreeing on what was "right" and without much exchange of thought.

The amount of time spent in consultation is important. How can a patient "reveal" so much of him- or herself in a five- or ten-minute interview? How long does it take for someone to design a kitchen or customize a wedding invitation or purchase a car? Should redesigning your face and body be any less exacting or meticulous?

Can cosmetic surgery be practiced without knowledge of the fifth dimension? Undoubtedly it can. In fact, this was primarily the case in the early days of cosmetic surgery when a Dr. X "performed" the exact same rhinoplasty on every patient (in fact, it might have been known as an "X rhinoplasty"), or when Dr. Y "did" a patient's face according to predetermined standard techniques, or when Dr. Z stated his favored approach to breast enhancement or reduction. Doctors were often known, and strived to be known, for a specific technique or post-operative look making their patients appear like so many factory products coming down the conveyor line.

This is not to say that these results were not "good" or acceptable. It just might not have been what a patient had envisioned. Often patients don't even know differently and to this day will ask, "What will I look like when I have…?" The appropriate question really should be, *"What do you need to do to give me what I want?"* Patients may not know all the options, possibilities, and variations to surgery, and thus not think to ask. They will assume the surgeon will know what will make them happy or they will simply accept what the surgeon gives them as what was possible. Surgery would have been performed, the patient might even have been happy, but the fifth dimension was not attained; it was merely stumbled upon. There must be a better approach. There must be more structure to the process.

You cannot practice plastic surgery responsibly without examining and interviewing the patients and probing them thoroughly. You cannot enter the fifth dimension without seeing the patients. You cannot get patients to a higher state of "happiness" (isn't that what they are after?) without the patients themselves knowing what will make them happy and stating that clearly to the plastic surgeon. I will encourage patients to tell me what they want, what they want to change, where they want to go, what will make them happy, what they dream of, and let me worry about if and how I can get them there.

Another very practical, and a most difficult, component of the fifth dimension is the understanding that the goal of the meeting of the minds is not necessarily, and not even often, the physical (i.e., anatomical) result, but is the psycho-emotional changes that occur. That is, it is not how big the breasts are, how tight the skin is, how flat the abdomen is, or how smooth the thighs are that count. Rather, it is how confident or content a patient feels, how attractive she imagines herself to be, and how normal she interprets her body shape to be. In addition, the body and face are constantly changing and so is the state of the patient's mind. Picasso did have it right. The body a person desires at twenty is not the body she cares about at sixty. The face she tries to enhance at thirty is not the worry she will have at seventy.

Often a patient will disrobe in front of a surgeon and, *without asking the patient a single question,* the surgeon might declare to the patient, "You need a..." The surgeon will assume she wants the tightest abdomen possible. He might imagine the maximum amount of fat suctioned. He will conjure up the plumpest lips, the most eye-catching breasts, or the most dramatic facial rejuvenation. The patient may want all these things... or she may not. The desire, the satisfaction, and the goal are in the patient's mind. That is where the secrets are kept and need to be unlocked. To this end, I often refer to what I do as *psychological surgery:* I operate on what one *sees* to affect what goes on between her ears and what she *thinks* and *feels.*

Attaining the fifth dimension is easily the most important, most challenging, most unpredictable, and most rewarding aspect to cosmetic surgery. It takes times, effort, introspection, and self-discovery. It is a rather elusive ideal to which I must strive. It requires sympathetic and discerning ears and eyes. It begins with the art of listening. But it will eventually reveal the most rational, logical, and customized course of action. It will guide my hands within the patient and lead my patient towards her ultimate, desired, and personalized goal.

CHAPTER 5:

A HEALTHY, STABLE, AND HAPPY LIFESTYLE

Question: What makes a candidate for cosmetic surgery?

Answer: A valid credit card.

* * *

Cosmetic surgery may not be necessary, but it is rampant. Everyone wants it. We all could use it. Many surgeons want to do it. Some think they can, especially those who don't. Non-surgeons and non-physicians practice it. A few are in jail for catering to the desires of the beauty-seekers and for unapologetically luring the uninformed. Desire and cash make it all too easy to throw open the operating room doors and patients will march themselves through if they can. So, dollar signs aside, when should patients have cosmetic surgery? What is the responsible answer?

Liposuction is one of the most requested surgical procedures, consistently in the top three in popularity, along with rhinoplasty and breast augmentation. Recent statistics compiled by our national plastic surgical societies report that over four hundred thousand liposuction operations are performed each year and over one billion, one hundred million dollars is spent on surgeon fees alone. Except for the emaciated, everyone has fat.

However, liposuction, as opposed to being a specific procedure, is merely a technique to selectively remove fat, usually through a small incision, with the assistance of a negative pressure vacuum or an energy source like laser or ultrasound. It can be used alone or in combination with other body-contouring procedures like abdominoplasty, brachioplasty (arm lifts), or breast reduction, each of which has multiple variations. Theoretically, almost everyone should be able to have liposuction. But when a patient comes in asking for liposuction, it doesn't mean it is appropriate or safe for her.

Currently, America has an obesity epidemic with two-thirds of the population either overweight or obese (defined as a body-mass index, BMI, expressed as kilograms of body weight/meters squared of height of over thirty). One would think that liposuction and other body-contouring procedures could be applied to virtually everyone, yet it is generally accepted among responsible plastic surgeons that these procedures are not the appropriate answer to obesity. Instead, the ideal candidate is typically someone who ironically may look like she does not need surgery and who is, according to some doctors, no more than twenty-five pounds from her ideal weight. Even then, the use of body-mass index to define obesity has been criticized as too simplistic. For example, high body-mass indices may be due to high muscle-mass content. Highly fit, but extremely muscular, athletes may be deemed obese based on this form of measurement. Absolute weight, weight relative to ideal, or BMI index all may not be good indicators of health, fitness, or appropriateness for body contouring. The question then is:

Who are the ideal patients and when are they optimal candidates for the procedure?

On the opposite side of the scale are patients who go through rapid weight loss through extreme dieting, superhuman exercise routines, or bariatric surgery. They subsequently look like they are dresses in search of a good tailor. Their faces and bodies are screaming for plastic surgery. Wrinkles and excess skin abound. Even the most skeptical might actually concur. Are they ready...and, if not, when?

* * *

For many years, I have advocated what I call "*a healthy, stable lifestyle*" for prospective patients contemplating body-contouring procedures. Just as the name suggests, body-contouring procedures are performed to alter the aesthetic shape of the body. While unpredictable secondary benefits may occur, such as reducing strain on the spine, helping treat diabetes and hypercholesterolemia, and controlling high blood pressure, these are not predictable and should not be promised or expected. The primary goal of body-contouring procedures is an enhanced appearance or visual effect that then translates into an improved quality of life and increased self-esteem. Common areas of concern are the breasts, the torso, and the lower extremities, but also the face, neck, and arms. While the same principle applies to all areas of cosmetic surgery, it is quite clearly demonstrated with body-contouring patients.

It is important to understand the mechanics of liposuction to understand when to best utilize it. Liposuction, in and of itself, is an extremely simplistic and safe technique and is one of the most common methods to contour the body. In its most popular form, a hollow cannula is attached to a vacuum device and a to-and-fro motion, whether manual or mechanized, pulls on the fat globules. Additional energy sources such as laser, powered water jets, radiofrequency, and ultra-sonic waves may be used as adjuncts to vaporize, emulsify, or implode fat cells. But there are inherent shortcomings, even dangerous elements, of these techniques when used on poor (i.e., poor as in inappropriate, such as obese, not necessarily financially disadvantaged) patients. The act of liposuction is often compared to picking grapes off the vines since clusters of fat cells are literally avulsed or torn or teased from their attachments. Ideally, this is done in a relatively gentle and selective manner such that only the grapes and not the vines, roots, or, God forbid, the entire lattice scaffolding are removed.

Since a tubular cannula is used to remove the fat cells, the cells are extricated from their three-dimensional space with a one-dimensional tool. Rows of fat cells are sucked out, leaving potential and real tunnels within that space. If carried to its extreme, the "space" left behind would consist of nothing but air and strands of connective tissue, nerves, and blood vessels; there would be little or no fat. The problem is that the tool is one-dimensional so the act of removing the fat is like trying to rake a sand box using a chopstick. It can be difficult to get the sand absolutely smooth unless you are a Buddhist monk with months of leisure at your disposal. If not applied uniformly, ripples, waviness, humps, and concavities can result. It doesn't matter if you use vacuum, laser, ultrasound, radio frequency, or water jet. Raking a beach is apt to be even more unsuccessful than raking a child's sand box, so limiting the surgical surface area is one of the key strategies to safely achieving a smooth result.

With the idea that suctioning of a small area of fat is inherently less risky than treating a large region, it is reasonable to conclude that the less liposuction you do in as small of an area as possible, the better and more predictable your result will be. A margin of error of 10 percent is only 10 cc's from a volume of 100 cc's, but it is 100 cc's from a volume of 1,000 cc's. So one goal, or requirement, is to limit the quantity and area of liposuction. Overweight or obese patients have a wider distribution of fat than healthy, fit patients and are therefore generally less ideal, or even inappropriate, candidates.

When applying liposuction, we are presumably removing the fat a patient does not want. That would be determined pre-operatively in consultation, usually with photos. Yet fat is necessary to the human body to support, protect, and separate the skin from underlying structures and to give the body aesthetic shape that is both natural and, hopefully, desirable. This means that there is fat that is intended to exist and should not be removed. This can be thought of as the "normal" fat. Conceptually, surgeons must determine what to remove and what to leave behind. A patient's wishful command of "Suck it out! Suck it all out!" should not be taken too literally. Being too aggressive at the sub-dermal level (where many of the small blood vessels feeding the skin live) can deprive the overlying skin of blood supply and cause skin necrosis. It can also remove the lubricating layer of fat that then causes deformities by allowing the skin to adhere unnaturally to the underlying muscles or bone.

If there is normal fat, there should be "abnormal" fat. By abnormal, I am not referring to fat that is diseased, but merely undesirable. Fat is not uniform. Fat in the face is not the same as fat around the intestines. Fat in the breast is not the same as fat on the abdomen. Some fat comes and goes easily. Normal fat metabolizes easily. But some fat stays until the bitter end. This is the "abnormal," "problem," or "undesirable" fat.

You cannot and should not remove all the fat everywhere. Some areas must remain "virgin" or untouched. This is the area considered normal and must be accepted by the patient and doctor as such. In effect, this area becomes the demilitarized zone where a cannula cannot invade. Therefore, another key goal is to identify and delineate the contour produced by "abnormal" fat, separating it from the "normal" fat. How and when is that done?

When an individual gains weight through increased fat, the contour will change according to the distribution of fat, the type of fat, and patient's genetics. Some women will see the change in their face. Some will see it in their hips. Others will see it in their breasts. Others will see it uniformly everywhere. Similarly, when a person loses weight by a decrease in fat, areas will diminish in size at different rates. I want to selectively remove fat to reveal a more pleasing shape.

It is very much like the metaphoric elephant joke:

Question: How do you sculpt an elephant?

Answer: Remove everything that doesn't look like an elephant.

It stands to reason that the most easily achieved and most *predictable* elephant sculpture is the sculpture that starts out looking most like an elephant. Philosophically speaking, I am trying to shape a person to uncover their true self. I want the patient to reflect, as closely as possible, what they think and feel about themselves. So how do I get the patient to look most like the person he or she wants to become *before* actually operating on them?

Diet and exercise are the standard answers. I know that when applied diligently and reasonably, diet and exercise will produce the most healthy and pleasing appearance for each individual patient. However, "diet" and "exercise" are not the important words; "individual" is.

There are probably more books written for the lay-public on diets and dieting than any other medical or health subject. A recent survey of Amazon.com revealed nearly 400,000 entries for all books on medicine, over 60,000 of them dealing with diets or dieting. Different diets have competing theories, some directly contradictory to one another. Diets seem to be as varied as the number of books in print. They often have good theories and seemingly reasonable rationale. But an American diet is not going to be meaningful for a Chinese person. A vegetarian diet is not going to be tolerated by a habitual carnivore. An Atkins diet may be difficult for a kosher family on vacation. Liquid diets will undoubtedly not last a lifetime. Nor will cookie diets. Home-delivered diets may not be affordable to a majority of the obese working class. Clearly, one diet, or even dieting in general, is not going to be helpful to many. Behavior, culture, finances, emotions, and genetics play too big a role to just send a patient out with "a diet."

Some people who are in tiptop shape are as thin as a rail with only 7 percent body fat. Others look equally good except for one or two pockets of annoying bulges such as "love handles" on men and "saddlebags" on women (why women don't call their fat "love handles" and men call theirs "saddlebags" is a mystery to me). Others will still be big and round like football centers. Ectomorphic, endomorphic, and mesomorphic describe inherent differences in body design and shape. *Fit and healthy people come in all shapes and sizes.*

At the opposite end of the spectrum, some people are categorized as morbidly obese with a BMI of over forty. Despite all their best intentions and efforts (by some reports, averaging twenty-four different diets), they will come to some bariatric surgery, such as gastric bypass, ileal jejunal bypass, or lap banding, to achieve significant weight loss.

When an overweight or obese person who looks like a great candidate for body-contouring procedures applies diet and exercise effectively, he starts to "lose" the excessive normal fat and leaves behind the abnormal or problem fat. (He doesn't actually lose the fat; it's just that the swollen fat cells shrink, divesting themselves of lipids.) The "real" person starts to emerge from under the fat and, while looking "better," the problem fat previously hidden among the overstuffed normal fat may begin to stand out and become more of a visual "problem." The person, as sculpture, starts to look like an imperfect elephant.

Ironically, the person is now a better candidate for body contouring, even though he has less body fat. There are obvious, well defined, and localized fatty regions. If the elephant looks like an elephant, then weight loss has done the work. If the sculpture looks sort of like an elephant except for a few bulges here and there, then it is easier, safer, and simpler to remove what doesn't look like an elephant. That is why plastic surgeons love to do liposuction on patients who don't even look like they "need" it. On the other hand, some patients can get more discouraged at this point because they continue to see the problem areas that have become more visually pronounced. They get frustrated by seeing less and less effect the more they work to lose weight. This is an opportune time for a plastic surgeon to step in before they overdo the dieting and exercise program.

Exercise will help mobilize the fat by increasing calorie expenditure, tone and increase the size of underlying muscles that form the deeper foundation of body contour, and make the cardiovascular system healthier. Reasonable patients understand and accept this requirement.

The problem sounds easy enough to solve. Diet and exercise. Exercise and diet. Easy to say. Hard to achieve. While I always encourage, even demand, that a prospective body-contouring patient maintain a good eating and exercise program, I am also aware that the recidivism rates with subsequent poor diet and lack of exercise are high. There are challenges to exercising that rival the challenges to dieting. Not everyone can, or will, spend three hours a day, or even an hour a day, five days a week, or even three days a week, every week, or even every other week, in the gym. Not everyone can tolerate riding a bicycle or walking on a treadmill. Similarly, not everyone will become vegetarians or stop eating desserts or fast foods or understand the ever-changing food pyramid. To ask this of them is fine, but unrealistic.

In fact, experts don't even agree on what a good diet plan is: high protein, low carbs, high carbs, low calories, low animal fat, three meal a day, six meals a day, unlimited meals, etc., etc. etc. Instead, what I ask of my patients is to maintain what I refer to as *their* "Individual Healthy and Stable Lifestyle."

While this approach is really undefined, curiously enough, most people know themselves, and know what is good and bad about their lifestyles. Those who don't know and don't care won't change anyway and should be approached surgically with extreme caution, if at all. *A prudent plan requires prudent participants. Responsible elective surgery requires responsible patients.* Tell a chronic beer drinker not to drink beer and he'll probably throw a six-pack at you. However, many people, and most prospective patients, will readily admit their sins: They like chocolates or they snack between meals or never exercise and don't like to play sports. They will even acknowledge certain illicit activities when pressed, like the occasional drag on a joint. They will complain about the time and energy demands of parenting but confess that even if they didn't have kids they wouldn't lift weights or play tennis. Knowing their own habits, patterns, or urges is a different matter than changing them, but it is an absolutely necessary first step.

While many people have the potential to become doctors, artists, executives, or teachers, not all will, nor need or should they. So-called human nature, that which encompasses drive, ambition, frustrations, motivations, and fears, and governs much of our behavior, tells us that we are individuals and will sink or rise to the levels that we determine for ourselves. We are all programmed to some extent to achieve or not achieve because of a multitude of factors, including our genetics, family backgrounds, cultures, peers, and life experiences. Some people relish a challenge while others run in the opposite direction. One person will take one talent and make ten and another will take ten and end up with one. Hope is ethereal, but liposuction is tangible, so the "normal" person will gravitate towards liposuction. The concept of sucking fat is easier to grasp. The ideal patient is a no-brainer. It is the less-than-ideal patient that will demand a rational strategy and philosophy.

Once patients acknowledge their lifestyle, they must ask themselves the hard and self-critiquing question of whether or not that lifestyle is healthy and whether or not it is sustainable. It does no good to work hard at something you do not enjoy doing in order to go through surgery that is otherwise unnecessary and then relapse back into an unhealthy lifestyle. Nor is it appropriate to know you have an unhealthy lifestyle but not care about improving it; that should automatically disqualify you from having elective cosmetic surgery. The goal for each individual patient is to *take the responsibility of putting themselves in the best possible lifestyle for their own health and peace of mind.* The fact that some of them might require a surgical solution to their obesity is not an excuse for not taking responsibility for their obesity. Understanding and taking responsibility is the goal, not just becoming thinner.

I learned as far back as the third year of Harvard Medical School that bad, as well as miraculous, things can happen in the operating room. While disease can be cured and lives saved in operating rooms, hemorrhage, infections, disfigurement, iatrogenic wounds, and strokes can also happen. You will never have a surgical complication if you never have surgery. You will never need secondary revision surgery if you never have a primary surgery. Patients must earn the right to enter the operating room and this is doubly so for "unnecessary" cosmetic surgery.

Operating room doors are too often left unlocked and flung wide open for inappropriate or marginal patients. Having a curable surgical condition, like appendicitis, is one way to "earn" the right, but what constitutes a right for the elective cosmetic surgery patient? Just having a padded bank account or good credit doesn't buy them the ticket, not in my practice. They must motivate themselves to work toward their potential, whether it is to make one talent two or ten. Once they make and achieve that pre-surgical commitment, God and nature, and perhaps their personal trainer, if they have one, will determine what they will look like.

A corollary to this is that the ultimate goal is to increase one's happiness and, therefore, the patient should be happy in adopting whatever lifestyle he or she chooses. Once the healthy, stable (and happy) lifestyle is achieved, then the plastic surgeon can go to work and see how close he can get to sculpting the elephant. Before that, it is like drinking wine before its time. The results will be sub-optimal and the patient and surgeon will have done themselves a disservice. I must constantly remind myself that some patients will still not be candidates for anything and some concerns cannot be improved no matter how much a patient desires it. Others will indeed become ideal candidates. And some will need to modify their expectations and elect other procedures or treatment strategies to suit their individual desires. Any patient who is able to make that commitment to herself will ultimately make better surgical choices, have fewer chances of complications, and end up with more accurate, predictable, and longer-lasting results.

If a patient becomes so motivated to achieve her healthy and stable lifestyle, she might forego surgery altogether. Just recently, a patient was due to undergo breast implant replacement. She began to inquire about liposuction of her hips, thighs, and buttocks. All of these areas were visibly disproportionate to the rest of her body. She was a mother of four and had neglected her own needs. She admitted that she was twelve pounds above her normal fighting weight and was always bothered by her lower torso. Since she was normally more active with tennis, treadmill, and running but had failed to maintain this exercise pattern, I explained the "Healthy, Stable Lifestyle" philosophy to her. She readily confessed her need to exercise more.

Six weeks later, just prior to her breast surgery, she happily revealed that she had resumed her exercise program, lost eleven pounds, and was less concerned about her hips, thighs, and buttocks. Furthermore, she had much more energy and felt much better about herself. Needless to say, she did not have the liposuction. I felt as satisfied as if I had done the surgery itself.

Yet another thirty-eight-year-old patient was pushing herself with an exercise program that stressed her knees and increased her frustration. The harder she worked out, the more pregnant she looked because of the resistant problem fat around her lower abdomen. A simple forty-five-minute operation using old-fashioned liposuction gave her the abdomen she worked so hard to attain. She was now healthy, stable, and happy!

Even more satisfying was the patient who came in five years after her abdominoplasty and liposuction and declared, "You changed my life, Dr. Yuan. After you talked to me about my lifestyle, I decided I had to get real and take care of myself." She started hiking again, doing Pilates, and eating healthier. With that, she had earned her ticket into the operating room.

Recent studies published in the *Journal of the American Medical Association* indicate that fitness (i.e., the "healthy" part of a healthy, stable lifestyle), as measured by baseline maximal treadmill exercise, was the predominant predictor of mortality of individuals over the age of sixty.[2] Fat content and obesity were less important than overall fitness. Fit individuals who were also obese were less likely to die than unfit individuals who were thin. This emphasis on fitness, and the subsequent healthy, stable lifestyle, corroborates my approach that the primary duty of plastic surgeons should be to look at the patient's lifestyle *before* judging fat content or body shape.

Now, let's get back to the definition of obesity and the issue of ideal versus normal weight. As a result of my emphasis on a healthy, stable (and happy) lifestyle, I really do not look too much at weight or even body-mass index (BMI) as a determinant of a patient's appropriateness for most cosmetic surgery procedures. There are a lot of genetic and uncontrollable factors that will affect a patient's weight. What I do look at is the *history* of their weight (i.e., the *change* or *stability* of weight over their fourth dimension of time).

Many people do not fit the usual actuarial charts plotting age, height, weight, and body mass. In fact,

2   Xuemei Sui et al., Cardiorespiratory fitness and adiposity as mortality predictors in older adults, *JAMA*, 2000; 298:2507-2516

current definitions and statistics on obesity are controversial. Absolute weight at a particular point in time is less informative than weight history over time. Even *weight* history may take a back seat to actual *contour* change in the anatomical areas of concern. For example, a patient inquiring about facial rejuvenation may be a reasonable surgical candidate if most of the fluctuation in weight is manifested elsewhere on her body and not in her face.

On the other hand, large swings (15 to 20 percent) within a relatively short period of time (i.e., less than a year) may be indicative of a relative contraindication for surgery if only as a barometer of the stability of a patient's lifestyle and habits. This is because these changes are significant and might override the contour changes the surgery is trying to influence. For example, a twenty-pound weight change will dwarf the effects of a five-pound liposuction. It is too much like trying to hit a moving target (or trying to sculpt a dodging elephant, as the analogy goes).

However, if a patient has been stable for a minimum of six months, preferably a year or more, and (this is a BIG "AND") he or she has a healthy lifestyle as far as diet, exercise activities, and habits are concerned, then an honest assessment of that patient can take place. This does not mean that any plastic surgery will be appropriate. It just means that it is fair to render judgment regarding the patient's appearance of body or facial contour at that particular point in time. There is no hard and fast rule or absolute cut-off in the queue into the operating room. But there definitely is an art to this science where judgment supersedes formulas. Bull's eyes are more easily hit when the target is clearly visualized and isn't moving all over the place.

While liposuction and abdominoplasties are the most common body-contouring procedures, obviously dependent on the healthy, stable lifestyle principle, breast procedures and facial rejuvenation procedures are also dependent on this prerequisite since fluctuations in weight might affect the size, shape, and contour of the breast and face, albeit usually to a lesser degree than the torso. One might adhere to this principle more or less strictly depending on the individual patient and her individual concerns.

The corollary to the truism that *the ideal cosmetic surgical candidate will have achieved a healthy, stable, and happy lifestyle* is *not every cosmetic concern has a good surgical solution.* Bad cellulite and stretch marks (or striae) are examples. Treatments are available but generally imperfect, if not ineffective. Recalcitrant obesity is another. Not every person has the potential to look like an Olympic athlete or celebrity. Even the celebrity does not look like the celebrity in person. Trust me on that one. Despite my own athletic endeavors, I am a prime example of one's limitations. Wishful thinking aside, I am just not *ever* going to have Matthew McConaughey's or Tiger Woods' physique. Not every person will earn the privilege of entering the operating room, even though some might feel they should be able to purchase this right in a free society with an America Express Platinum Card.

By achieving and maintaining a healthy and stable lifestyle, the doors will unlock and open a little wider by clarifying what can and cannot be done surgically. You should not be able to buy, or talk, or plead, or force, or cry your way into an operating room for an elective cosmetic procedure.

Because of their failure to attain, and adhere to, a healthy, stable lifestyle, not all patients will be good surgical candidates. It is also just as true that operating on patients who have definitely *not* achieved a healthy, stable lifestyle is inviting complications and suboptimal or unstable results in spite of perfect execution of technique. Recently, a plastic surgeon was being crucified in the media for a string of bad results and disfiguring complications. In a display of profound denial and arrogance, he answered the criticism of this slew of surgical complications resulting in malpractice suits with the statement that he was not at fault. He explained that there wasn't any problem with the surgeries he performed; it was just that the patients were poor surgical candidates to begin with. Huh??? **Choosing the appropriate patient is more important than performing a surgical technique perfectly.**

* * *

To me, much, if not all, of what plastic surgery is about is getting at the truth. Each patient is, in small part, like a patient undergoing transgender transformation. When a man feels like a woman but looks like a man, or vice versa, plastic surgery can reconcile the outer manifestation with their inner feelings. The same is true to some lesser, but no less important, extent with a woman who feels young but looks old. Or one who feels sensual, but doesn't see sensuality in her body. Or a teenager that wants to feel normal but doesn't look it because his ears stick out too far or her nose is crooked or hangs too low. You have to use truth to find the truth. The healthy, stable lifestyle model is a way for patients to accept truths about themselves without ostracism or belittlement. It substitutes factual judgment for emotional judgment. It is not imposed truths or someone else's truth. It is one's own truth. You don't have to compare yourself to another individual or an idealized chart. A person knows when he is not exercising enough or when his eating habits are not healthy. She knows when she has met her limitations and when she has tried or not tried diligently to find them. He knows what he enjoys doing and what no one can ever get him to do.

You can tell a person that she is attractive, but if she doesn't feel or believe it herself, it won't be the truth to her. Only when a person acknowledges the shortcomings in her lifestyle can she then begin to take measures to correct or improve on them. As in addictive personalities, *self-revelation is the key to cure.* When a person realizes his or her potential and accepts his or her limitations, then an honest assessment of the benefits of plastic surgery can take place. The truth is that there are things that plastic surgery *can* change, some things plastic surgery *can't* change, some things *only* plastic surgery can fix, and some things that plastic surgery *shouldn't* fix. The challenge and the task for both plastic surgeon and patient are to discern one from the other. And that is the truth.

As well as assisting in reconciling the outer person with the inner, plastic surgery truly has the power to change people from the inside out if each patient is forced to adopt the healthiest and most stable lifestyle he or she is capable of. Many of my patients have willed themselves off of cigarettes and have managed to stay off because of their desire to have some plastic surgery. Some patients have never exercised in their life but will now walk at least a few times a week. Some have rewarded themselves with plastic surgery after totally transforming their lifestyle by becoming active, responsible, and happy human beings. The hope and goal is that once patients have worked hard to open the doors to the operating room, earned the right and privilege of entering that operating room, and spent time, money, and effort having the cosmetic plastic surgery they desire, their lifestyle will have then changed for the better.

CHAPTER 6:

THERE'S NO SUCH THING AS BEST

"You are THE BEST!"
       —What all plastic surgeons love to hear

* * *

How many times have I and every other plastic surgeon heard those words? We want to believe. We need to believe. So we do.

Smiling with feigned modesty and puffing out my chest a bit, I say—to myself, of course—"Yes, I am The Best."

I've had the best education, been to the best schools, survived the best medical and surgical training, benefited from the best mentors, and been blessed with the best parents. I certainly own the best car, live in the best neighborhood, am a citizen of the best country in the world, and, without a doubt, have the best kids in the universe. By the way, earth is the best planet in the best solar system in the best universe. Who can argue with all this? I am the product of The Best.

It brings to mind a patient who, on the day he shuffled into my office, was probably the most recognizable rock singer in the world. Bolstered by the confidence-building comment his doctor gave him that "Dr. Yuan's the best," he stated he wanted me to do a facelift, apparently his third. He said it almost matter-of-factly, as if he needed another hi-amp speaker on stage. But I know that whenever a high-profile patient comes to me after having surgery elsewhere, I can be assured of an interesting story. He had his previous surgeries with a highly publicized plastic surgeon some ten years ago whose other celebrity patients had no reservations about letting the world know about their cosmetic adventures. While celebrities are not widely known to have surgery with necessarily the most highly reputable plastic surgeons (in fact, it can be quite scary whom some do go to), his former surgeon was quite a formidable and respected technician. It was obvious that someone who had once been "The Best" in this rocker's mind had fallen out of favor and now I was taking his place. Mr. Rocker was used to having the best of everything: a mansion in Beverly Hills, a castle in England, a beach house in Malibu.

"Personally," he bluntly announced in his English accent, "I think he was on something." Who, if not Mr. Rocker himself, should know?

Me? Being called The Best isn't always what it is cracked up to be.

* * *

Do what you think is best, doc. Use the best implant. Give me the best result you can. Do the best operation there is. What is the best?

The concept of "best" seems self-evident and simple. Since things are not the same, one thing should be better than another. If followed to its logical conclusion, there should be a best. In fact, there should be nothing but the best. That is the foundation of capitalism. The cream rises to the top. The weak (i.e., those who are not the best) do not survive. Evolution is competition and adaptation, creating better products and a better species. It seems one can't have a worst without there being a best. Life is all about doing, achieving, getting, and rewarding the best: Darwinian at its best.

The problem is...**there is no such thing as best.** And I tell my patients exactly that.

When I make that bold statement surrounded by my degrees from the best educational institutions in the world, patients look lost, as if I just told them that their grocery store doesn't sell food and I don't know where else to look. They are spending precious moments with me because of some recommendation or a reputation that they believe is worth their time, effort, and money. People may have a limit on their financial resources, but no one intuitively wants anything but the best for themselves or their loved ones. Imagine if your doctor said he was going to recommend something less than the best thing for you.

"Here, I've decided that I'm going to perform a second-rate operation. It's not quite The Best thing, but it's the next best thing."

"The Best? Why would you want The Best? This'll be good enough."

"Ha! If you wanted The Best, you shouldn't have come here. You won't find any Best here."

No one wants to hear that they do not rate or are not receiving the best...even if they aren't. I certainly want the best for my patients, as do most self-respecting doctors, just as we want what is best for our children and loved ones. Yet it is not always, in fact rarely, clear as to what is the best for any particular patient, certainly not after a ten- minute consultation.

This decision dilemma is not unique to plastic surgeons. It is not solely the function of plastic surgery as an artistic profession: the art-is-in-the-eye-of-the-beholder quandary. It is a logical conclusion to an analytical situation that is a result of multiple variables, all of which are non-comparable or, at best (pardon the pun), non-quantifiable: the apple-versus-orange predicament. And it is inherent to the practice of medicine. How can one really compare a painful but quick surgery to a painless, drawn-out medical treatment? How would we rate a 5 percent risk of life-threatening infection with a 2 percent risk of paralysis? Which is worse, hardening of a silicone gel implant or leakage of a saline implant? Which is best, a surgeon who has done the same operation a thousand times or one who can improvise and innovate a unique surgical solution to a difficult problem?

The undeniable, and contrary, truism is that all surgeries carry a host of risks and promise a variety of attributes, and cannot often be strictly compared to each other at all. If a procedure is riskier but its result lasts longer, is it necessarily better than a simple operation that doesn't last as long? That is basically the battle between more complicated facial rejuvenation surgery and less invasive "quick fixes." With cosmetic surgery, there is also the ambiguous and infinitely variable element of taste or visual perception or emotional response: It is whatever you want to call that "thing" that permits, or forces, us to discern good from not so good, attractive from unattractive, desirable from undesirable.

Magazines and consumer guides are always naming the best car or truck of the year. They often have a complex grading system with a whole committee of experts. They rate everything from fuel efficiency to turning radius to cargo capacity to rear passenger comfort. Often, any proclamation itself can produce a self-fulfilling prophecy whereby the best-car-of-the-year accolade influences the public to buy that car and the public then declares it the best car because who wants to drive a car that is not The Best? That certainly happens with any consumer product, including plastic surgery treatments and procedures. Everyone would then buy the one and only best. But they don't. And that is because every consumer, like every plastic surgery patient, has individual desires, individual needs, individual tastes, individual financial resources, individual fears, and so on. A cursory survey of an airline magazine revealed no less than four different "best steakhouses in America" lists. Not only is there a variety of cars and trucks, sneakers, and pain medications, there is even a variety of Supreme Beings one can choose from: God, Allah, Mohammed, Jesus Christ, Brahman, Confucius, maybe even L. Ron Hubbard!

A very common practical example is a patient who comes in seeking breast enlargement. Unfortunately, for some plastic surgeons, once a woman utters the words "breast enlargement" or "breast implants," an operation and a specific look comes to mind: round, perky, C-cup, 320 cc's. Within ten seconds or less, the surgeon can have the whole procedure blocked out and the patient can find herself sitting in front of a surgical consultant or "closer" (just like in baseball) being told how fabulous she will look. After all, the doctor is The Best and the patient has already told the doctor to do what he thinks is Best. So he does.

But one Best surgeon will use a high-profile implant and another Best surgeon will use a moderate-profile implant. One will use a textured implant while his colleague will use smooth. Another will opt for a shaped implant while his cross-town competitor will choose a round one. Each of them will honestly believe he has used The Best.

Often a patient will shop around and get multiple opinions. Each doctor comes with some feather in his cap or has some qualification to deserve recommendation; in twenty years of private practice, I have had only a handful of patients come to me "off the street" without a personal referral. A visit to four different Best surgeons can buy a patient five different Best opinions. One tip-off to judge if the Best surgeon believes he has a Best approach would be to ask how he or she performs a specific procedure. A definitive, unwavering response can be read as an affirmation for the "best" procedure: "I *always* do it this way" or "My technique is such-and-such because it gives me the best results."

The breast augmentation procedure has about six major variables plus the irreproducible variable of technical skill and the variable of post-surgical healing with all of its many components of swelling, bruising, neurosensory re-innervation, scar contraction, soft tissue "give," and muscular relaxation. I typically take three to four sessions over a minimum period of two to three weeks to sift through nearly a hundred different operations with the patient, finally coming up with an operation derived from the patient's own choosing that is not necessarily The Best for everyone.

First, there is the incision. There are four potential incision sites: transaxillary, periareolar, inframammary, and transumbilical. All have advantages and disadvantages and, thus, the many choices. It is not clear that one is better than the other but that one may make the procedure easier or safer. One may produce a less conspicuous scar while another may have a lower risk of poor healing. For different patients, a different incision will be used.

While there are statistics on acceptability rates on certain scars, the fact is one cannot predict with any accuracy how a particular scar in a particular patient will turn out. In fact, one can have a "good" scar on one breast and a "bad" scar on the other. Even more perplexing is the presence of "skip" areas where a scar will be alternately "good" or "bad" along the same incision. My advice to patients has been to not think about where they want a good scar, since by definition it is good, but perhaps where they don't want a bad scar. All things being equal, that might tip them towards or away from a particular location.

Second, there is the position of the implant. Generally speaking, you can put the implant on top of the chest wall muscles, so-called *subglandular* since the implant is under the breast gland. This is where the breast normally resides so the implant may move and sit more naturally; exotic dancers and body-builders typically have implants placed subglandular. Or, you can place it under the chest wall muscles, so-called *submuscular* for obvious reasons. Normally, there is nothing under the muscles except for the ribs so it is an unnatural, but effective, location. Since the implants can distort during muscle activity, body-builders tend to not have implants placed sub-muscular. But for some unknown reason (there are many theories), submuscular implants tend to have a lower risk of capsular contracture or hardening. So which location is The Best?

Next is the choice of implants. If we had to opt between a saline implant or a silicone implant, we would need to decide if it is best to have a better chance at a natural feel to the breast (silicone gel) or a lower risk of significant capsular contracture or hardening (saline). Saline implants, because the filler material is simply salt water and is liquid in consistency, start out a little firm (like a water balloon) but have a lower risk (5 to 10 percent) of hardening to the point of distortion (grade 3) or pain (grade 4). Silicone implants can be virtually undetectable by feel at the outset because of their gelatinous quality, but may have up to a 30 to 50 percent risk of significant hardening in the future.

Is it better to know when an implant is leaking, as when a saline implant collapses, or to have an implant that one doesn't even know is leaking, such as can occur with silicone gel implants? Is it better to have to buy another operation because an implant deflates (saline) or possibly live the rest of your life without suspecting that the implant has leaked because everything looks and feels fine (silicone gel)? Saline, silicone, silicone, saline...

Once we make that decision, we must choose the characteristics or style of the implant bag. Should it be smooth or textured, round or shaped? Some doctors only use smooth implants. Some doctors only use textured. Does it matter? Which is best? If there is some doctor who is using each of the different types of implants available, does it matter what is used since obviously each doctor believes he or she is using the best implant? Can there be multiple "Bests" and thus no one "Best"? Is "Best," then, a misnomer?

Finally, the one thing that can, as I like to say, "blow everything else out of the water" is the size. An implant that holds a volume of 150 cc's is vastly different than a 350-cc implant. And a 350-cc implant in a 150-cc breast is going to impact the breast more than a 150-cc implant in a 350-cc breast or a 350-cc implant in a 350-cc breast. In breast implants, size is truly relative. As I explain it to my patients, how important an implant will be is determined by the relative amount of the final breast that is implant and the amount that is natural breast. If I put a pea-sized implant into a large breast, it doesn't matter what kind of implant it is; it will act and feel like the natural breast. But if I put a humungous implant into a flat breast, how the breast will look, act, and feel will be almost *entirely* determined by the type of implant.

Nowadays, size is usually measured in base diameter or implant width. A 300-cc implant with a base diameter of thirteen centimeters is going to produce a different breast than a 300-cc implant with an eleven-centimeter base diameter. An implant with a base diameter of eleven centimeters may hold anywhere from 200 cc's to 240 cc's to 320 cc's, depending on the profile or projection. The size by volume is a byproduct of the base diameter and projection. Plastic surgeons no longer refer to implants by volume, but by base width, style, profile, and manufacturer. Is it better to be large or **large** or **LARGE**? Is an implant with a wider base diameter better or worse than one with a narrower base diameter?

As we change decisions at every step of the operation-building process, the end result will change. When one decision is made, this might impact another decision. For example, if a patient with a small breast wants to go much larger, the base diameter of the required implant may or may not give her the volume increase she is looking for. As she increases the volume of the implants, a round implant may produce a breast that is too round for her tastes and require looking at shaped implants. Or, if she increases the width of the implant, she will start to see the outline of the implants beyond the borders of her natural breast and perhaps see or feel more rippling. Concern with rippling might dictate the use of silicone, rather than saline, implants. One Best choice may affect another Best choice. How are we assured that we will end up with the overall Best Choice? Choosing the Best Appetizer, the Best Entrée, the Best Dessert, and the Best Beverage may not guarantee the Best Meal. The only thing we can guarantee is that we won't end up hungry eating a horrible meal and that we have made honest and reasonable choices.

Injectable fillers are quite the rage now. Yet there are well over a hundred different materials in different forms and variable consistencies available. Some are longer-lasting. Some are softer. Some are more biocompatible. Some are biodegradable while others are permanent. Some produce fewer side effects. But none are perfect substitutes for what we need and none is the same as what nature and God gave us to begin with. Even what nature and God gives us is imperfect—otherwise, we wouldn't need injectable fillers. When cosmetic patients say they want to look natural, I tell them they already look natural, they just don't like it. We pick our poison (sometimes literally, as in the case with Botox).

The absence of an absolute and ultimate operation or technique is one of the most difficult truisms for a patient to grasp and to come to terms with, yet it is also the reason doctors may state what they believe is the best: Patients crave it. Patients come in with the inherent idea that they are going to get definitive answers to their quest for The Best procedure. While they nod in agreement with my reasoning for the disappointing explanation, there is a morbid resignation that is so hard to accept, like knowing one is never going to win the lottery or Nobel prize or go to Harvard University or get a date with George Clooney or Jennifer Aniston—even less likely, all of the above. It is just not going to happen. But once they embrace the concept, like life is finite and money isn't everything, the decision-making process becomes much clearer, logical, and less stressful. One can focus on what one truly wants, tempered with, and guided by, constraints of reality.

One of the most problematic and stressful aspects to decision-making is not necessarily deciding what the right choice is; there are many appropriate and reasonable choices. But it is *the fear of making a wrong choice.* Being right and not being wrong are not synonymous. It is like picking stocks. We can all pick stocks that have a reasonable chance of performing well. But we all are handicapped by the possibility of picking a stinker and losing real money. Faced with the challenge or necessity of picking the very Best stock, and putting our fortunes and reputations on the line, we crumble; we either don't pick any stocks at all or defer the responsibility of the choice to others.

Some of us may remember the enthusiasm of trying to answer questions in school mixed with the anxiety of raising our hands in class and having self-doubts about giving the right answer. Many children end up not raising their hands because of this insecurity and allow less smart but more self-confident, hardier students to sacrifice their egos with the wrong answer. Being wrong can have real consequences. Choosing a life partner for ourselves or projecting a life path for our children can produce similar anxiety and self-doubt.

Most patients find it easier to allow the plastic surgeon to make decisions for them. The patients may or may not be able to make a decision on their own, but they trust that the doctor has the right answer and certainly won't give them a wrong answer. They assume the doctor will in fact give them The Best answer and are happy to abdicate that role. Even after discussing how important it is for them to express their own desires and have their own opinions about their options, most patients will still ask, "So what do *you* think, doc? What would *you* do?"

The liberating corollary to the fact that there is no Best among valid choices is that one cannot make a wrong choice, and certainly not The Worst choice. You can make bad choices. You can make unwise choices. You can make more expensive or more painful choices. You can make an uninformed choice. But if you are responsible and sane, and you have the facts, you cannot make wrong choices.

I sense that when I tell patients that there is no Best choice and there are no wrong choices, they either have anxiety that is incompatible with undergoing plastic surgery (because they truly believe that there *must* be a best operation and will be disappointed, even angry, when they later find out that there was no such thing as Best or that they didn't get The Best), or they experience calmness knowing that as long as they make honest choices and understand the consequences, they cannot be wrong. After all, life is about making choices at the time you have to make them. Making a *better* choice with the advantage of hindsight is just not reality. Like in a marriage that goes awry, the bride or groom you pick is not necessarily the wrong spouse. She or he just *became* the wrong one. At the time, it probably seemed like the best choice.

In a creative endeavor like plastic surgery, the concept of, and the striving for, the ultimate, perfect, Best goal is inherent. Consciously or subconsciously, we are trying to better what is natural. We are trying to improve, not diminish. We are always lifting up— eyelift, facelift, neck lift, mid-facelift, breast lift, body lift—*never* pulling down. We are trying to create, not destroy. We are trying to increase self-esteem, not decrease it. Everything is geared toward better, and better, and better, until we hopefully attain The Best.

Nearly all doctors truly feel they are delivering the best treatment for their patients. So is it really important to determine if there truly is a best, an absolute Best, as long as there is a *perception of the best?* For many, it doesn't matter because they trust their doctors. It becomes a moot point or rather merely an experiment in intellectual discussion. In fact, as opposed to necessary medical treatment that treats an abnormality or pathology, cosmetic surgery as unnecessary medicine treats a perceived abnormality. It is probably more important and relevant when something goes wrong and you wonder in retrospect whether you made the best choice. But if you're happy, you're happy. The choice you made becomes The Best. You don't care about the other choices, like you don't care about other potential spouses if you are happily married. If you're not happy, you try to find out why you are not and what you can do to be happy. Maybe only then you realize that the choices you made were not "The Best."

Yet if we accept the fact that there is no such thing as best, we cannot know if we have actually attained it. The patient with the smooth implant thinks she has gotten the best. The patient with the textured implant thinks she has the best. Both of them are right until something goes wrong and then they believe they didn't get the best. But up until that point, each might believe she received the best, not really knowing what it is like to have the other patient's implant. It is highly unlikely that a patient will live in a vacuum and never come in contact with other patients. The only way to be truly satisfied is to make honest choices and to know and accept the premise that there is no such thing as Best. No operation is a hundred percent successful.

I have seen patients get ensnared in a vicious, destructive, and expensive game of what I call "*Chasing the Imperfection.*" This is most often the case with breast augmentation because what the patient is dissatisfied with is what is natural and "God-given"—yet still unacceptable—and what she is using to improve is manmade and thus fallible. The same is often the case with scars that are natural sequelae of a body's tendency to close a wound and keep it closed but that are, at times, incompatible with social definitions of beauty.

The way the game is played is the patient must believe that there is such a thing as "Best" and is in constant pursuit of "The Best," where she gets everything she desires without any side effect or complication. A substantial entry fee is required to enter the game. As she experiences some inherent side effect or imperfection or dissatisfaction from her Best surgery, she finds it difficult to believe that she has indeed attained "The Best." Guilt, blame, sorrow, regret, and anger can creep in. Then in an effort to capture the real "Best," she antes up another entry fee and undergoes some other treatment that, while intended to treat the imperfection, has some other imperfection as a byproduct. Another entry fee is sacrificed and another round of "Chasing the Imperfection" ensues. Now the patient is convinced that she is not in possession of "The Best" and is even more intent on pursuing it.

As the saying goes in plastic surgery, the enemy of good is better. Here the enemy of better is best. Or as my father used to put it, "Don't be worried about what you don't have. Be happy with what you do." There is no such thing as "best."

The question of who is the best or what makes the best plastic surgeon is a common query among prospective patients and the lay-audience. Publications love printing the "Best" lists. Doctors love these when they are on them, though it is impossible to compare all the plastic surgeon against each other. Most "Best Lists" these days have some bias or quid-pro-quo. We all want to believe we are *among* the best. Recently I was "nominated" to a "Top Ten in Beverly Hills" list only to be asked to pay a fee to be publicized as such. While it is truly reassuring and humbling to be named to the "Best of…" lists and to be honored with a patient's enthusiastic, if not misplaced, adulation as "The Best," it is not because I believe it is true. In fact, patients with body dysmorphic disorder who are poor candidates for cosmetic surgery often will attempt to win a doctor over by such extreme flattery. But in my own odd form of insecurity, I am relieved to know that I am certainly not the "Worst," most likely one of the "Better," and that patients will not make a "wrong" decision by coming to me. Usually I'll just smile, nod to them, and think quietly to myself, *There's no such thing as best.*

CHAPTER 7:

IT'LL LAST AS LONG
AS YOU WANT

"Forever is a long, long time"
　　—Big Mama *(The Fox and the Hound 1981)*

"Nothing is forever"
　　—Arnold Henry Glasow, American humorist

* * *

No one wants to go through cosmetic plastic surgery over and over again. In that, it is similar to marriage. One looks for lifelong bliss with little thought of failure or a reluctant return to the altar.

Of course, many newlyweds are fearful or realistic enough to ask themselves, probably in the privacy of their own thoughts, while pinning on a boutonniere or adjusting the veil or even at the very moment the rings appear, "Is this going to last?" But even then, I doubt we ("we" because I was once married) expect that the marriage will only last for a finite period of time. We don't hope to get five or ten or twenty years from marriage (although in today's world with all its freedom of travel, variety of lifestyles, and improved life expectancies, I could make an argument for ten-year marriage vows renewable every five to ten years by mutual consent). We don't expect happiness only until the kids turn eighteen or one of our AARP memberships kicks in. We hope we are blessed with a lifetime of joyful matrimony—"forever and ever" or "until death do us part."

There are numerous fields of study dealing with the failure of marriage and the disintegration of the family. An entire industry is devoted to the prevention, processing, and disposal of divorce. Similarly, much of plastic surgery and many plastic surgeons' entire careers are founded on the principle of failure. We try to improve techniques to limit the risk of failure because we all experience failure (failure not only in not being successful, but also not lasting forever). Some surgeons become experts in secondary procedures (re-dos, revisions, salvages, touch-ups) because of failed primary procedures. Secondary surgery is expected, even planned for, but not always because of outright failure. Despite known revision rates of 5 to 20 percent and higher in liposuction, rhinoplasty, and breast augmentation surgery, and despite a 50 percent divorce rate after first marriages and 60 percent after second, people still flock to these life-altering events.

Prospective breast augmentation patients routinely question the longevity of implants. Many accept the prevailing misconception that implants need to be changed every ten years or so. That, of course, is not true. What is true is that implants are known to have problems, one of which is leakage, and that the incidence of leakage is closely related to the length of implantation; the longer you have had an implant, the more probable that it will leak at some point in time. The manufacturers know this. There is money set aside in the form of warranties to pay for this. Doctors know this. We plan for it and advise patients of it. In some studies, second generation silicone gel implants were found to have a leakage rate exceeding 50 percent when implanted for more than ten years.[3, 4] Because of the fear and potential dangers of silicone gel outside its intended bag, the notion of routine replacement as a prophylactic measure arose. It's just playing the odds; replace the implants before the odds of leakage exceed the odds of non-leakage.

This, however, does not apply to saline implants, the content of which is simply sterile saline solution, an innocuous fluid. Here, we can wait until the leak actually occurs. But before we can recommend *routine* replacement of silicone gel implants, we need to ask what the dangers of a ruptured silicone gel implant really are. If the saline implants leak, they obviously did not last. But if the silicone implant is replaced before it leaks, can we say the surgery didn't last? Can a patient's fear of implants not lasting contribute to the impermanence of the same implants?

Another known fact is that implants do develop problems that make them function less than ideally, even though they do not leak. Capsular contracture, or hardening of the implant due to scar tissue shrinking around the implant, can distort the appearance of the implant and make for painful or firm breasts that are bothersome to the patient. (Because walling off an implant is what a body is designed to do, it is

3 Among others, Donna L. de Camara, Sheridan, J.M., and Kammer, B.A., Rupture and Aging of Silicone Gel Breast Implants, *Plast. Reconstr. Surg.* 91(5): 828-834, 1993.
4 Rod J. Rohrich et al., An Analysis of Silicone Gel-filled Breast Implants: Diagnosis and Failure Rates, *Plast. Reconstr. Surg.*, 102(7):2304-2308, 1998

surprising that all implants do not get hard.) Visible or palpable rippling, caused by waviness of the implant bag as it rests on the chest, can be embarrassing to the patient. Because the implants in these two situations are not functioning optimally, a patient can say that the procedure has failed or is unsuccessful in achieving an intended goal. In this sense, the implants might not be acceptable and the surgery might be said not to have lasted, especially if the patient decides to remove or exchange the implant.

Achieving an end result and being happy with the end result are not the same things. We all have purchased things in life or had expectations of events—a movie, a vacation, a date—that did not fulfill our expectations no matter how much we anticipated them. Some patients will be satisfied with fulfilling some, but not all, of the expectations. They are the glass-half-full types. They are happy with "better" and do not need "best." Surgical results will probably last longer for these patients.

Statistics in many studies showed that a high percentage of breast augmentation patients undergo a second surgery within five to ten years. But what is not widely known among the lay-public is that many of these secondary procedures are not related to failure of the implant, but to the desire of the patient. They want bigger, or smaller, breasts, have had pregnancies and require breast lifts or reductions, or are just unhappy with the shape or feel of the implants.

Because there is no such thing as the best implant, a patient with one type of implant may dislike one characteristic, such as rippling, and opt to change it to another type of implant, while the patient with the second type of implant may be unhappy with a different characteristic, such as roundness, and elect to change the implant to the first type. You can go round and round and not find anything that works perfectly. A Ferrari is not a better car than a Rolls Royce (and I have neither); it is just faster. And a Mercedes is not better than a Honda (and I have both); it is just more expensive. Even with the choices between silicone and saline implants, neither is better than another. It depends on how you use them and what criteria or characteristic you are measuring. In many respects, short of leakage, the breast augmentation patient herself controls how long the surgery will last.

Some procedures are unequivocal failures either by flawed design or poor execution. Traditional mini-facelifts were disappointing to many. Eventually, among plastic surgeons, the reputation of the mini-facelift was "mini-lift, mini-result." Thread lifts using barbed sutures also did not hold up under scrutiny. These catered to patients who didn't want to go through, or couldn't afford, the "real" facelift. The same was true for some of the modern resurfacing technologies using non-ablative modalities, whether they were lasers, radio frequency, or ultrasound energy. Patients often saw no to minimal improvement with their skin. There is little argument that these particular results did not last.

Facelift patients who opt for the "full" lift also ask how long surgical results will last. This is even trickier. With a facelift, there is nothing that will mark a definitive failure except disastrous complications like skin necrosis and nerve damage. With a breast implant, it fails when it leaks. With a hip replacement, it fails when it breaks or gets infected. With a tire, it fails when it goes flat. While a facelift does not break, there can be a time when it loses its intended effect. How long will it take to do so? Of course, that is dependent on two things; the first is the reason one does the facelift in the first place, and the second is what the patient thinks about the first factor.

The reason someone has a facelift can be as concrete as removing the sagging, the so-called turkey gobbler or waddle, under the neck. If that is accomplished, the facelift technically is a success. However, even if the sagging is gone, the patient may still not be satisfied. Conversely, despite some residual sagging, a patient may consider surgery a success if she feels better about herself. If the sagging is not changed at all, or very little, one can safely conclude that most patients would consider the surgery unsuccessful, placebo effect notwithstanding.

If we assume that the facelift is technically a success and that the projected anatomical changes are achieved, how long does this physical state last? When will results start to regress? While plastic surgeons search for and argue about facelift techniques that give longer-lasting effects, there is no consensus on the "right way" to perform a long-lasting facelift. In fact, a "facelift" itself is an antiquated term (as explained later) and may be used in a generic sense by both doctor and patient. There are actually many variations on the theme.

On the other hand, the reason to do a facelift might be very ill-defined. Perhaps it is to feel better about oneself or to look younger. Then it might "fail" when the patient no longer feels better or no longer looks young despite what she actually looks like.

Thus, the longevity of a procedure can be judged based on an *anatomical* change, a *cognitive* perception of an anatomical change, or an *emotional* assessment of an anatomical change. They are not the same things. Is there a change? Can you see the change? How do you feel about the change? Defining, separating out, and agreeing on each are at the heart and soul of cosmetic surgery.

While the adage "nothing lasts forever" is applicable to plastic surgery, there is value in knowing how long the post-surgical anatomic change will last. Patients want to know. Doctors want to know. Spouses want to know. The person paying the surgeon's fee wants to know. The answer is: We don't really know.

Each patient will have a different physical characteristic regarding skin elasticity, quantity of skin, volume (or its lack) of fat, and bony structure. Each component will impact the weathering of the tissues by gravity and time. We can get hints from the progression of a person's face through time (the fourth dimension). I always ask the patient to bring in photos from preceding decades to analyze how she ages. Some develop wrinkles from *loss of elasticity* and others have perceived sagging because of *loss of facial fat.* But that is retrospective analysis, not prospective prediction. It only tells us how the patient got to where she is, not where she might be going. These two aging patterns are treated differently with different types of facial rejuvenation techniques.

In reviewing progressive family photos, familial patterns may be evident. But familial patterns may justify a certain feature of a person, not predict the aging process for this unique individual in that particular family. For example, individuals will show signs of aging at different intervals of life. We all know people who have aged "prematurely" and others who have aged "gracefully"; these two patterns of aging may even occur within the same family. Likewise, if plastic surgeons cannot reliably predict how a person will age *before* surgery, how can we predict how she will age *after* surgery? After all, a patient's aging continues unabated and is superimposed upon whatever surgical changes take place. The only thing we can say with relative assurance is that if we "correct" the characteristics (i.e., sagging, wrinkling, loss of or excess fat) that produced the aged look, then the patient should look less aged in the future with the surgery than without.

However, even this seemingly obvious conclusion has caveats, as plastic surgeons have learned from past experience with lower lid fat removal, facial liposuction, and certain specific face-lifting techniques. While reversing the perceived causes of aging, immediate post-operative effects and long-term effects can later produce a strange, gaunt, or even cadaveric appearance, giving patients a more aged look. Then some surgeon will be doing secondary procedures to correct the primary procedure's shortcomings or side effects. Was the wrong procedure performed or did the results just not "last"?

The cognition of the anatomical changes and the emotional response to these changes are even more important. What does the patient think? This is the fifth dimension of plastic surgery as art. The patient will consciously or subconsciously respond psycho-emotionally to the end result once the healing is effectively complete. Subtle changes can be like achieving Nirvana while dramatic changes can be devastating. As plastic surgeons, we can have satisfaction or disappointment in obtaining the end result we envisioned as a test of our own surgical and artistic abilities. But we have to keep our own fingers crossed behind our backs while awaiting the patient's *response* to the results. Patients and doctors do not always agree on the effectiveness of the end results. As with unveiling a piece of art for the first time, plastic surgeons hold their breath for signs of the patient's first reaction. Our reaction to the patient's response can be as healing or destructive as good or bad surgery itself. Sometimes we have to temper a patient's enthusiasm while at other times we have to mollify their initial disappointment or anxiety. Like with great golfers, course management and controlling emotions can be the difference between winning and losing.

Beyond this second factor of patient response is the fact that the individual patients are complex and dynamic beings influenced by more than just what they see at the surgical site. All aspects of their life as thinking, feeling human beings come into play from continued concerns about age or beauty, interpersonal relationships, internal battles between self-esteem and confidence, self-interest and guilt, to financial conditions, sexual activities, or social calendars. Patients can initially love a result then grow to be dissatisfied or they can be traumatized by the loss of self then adapt and become ecstatic.

A comment from a spouse or friend, or even a stranger, can cause a patient to go from fan to critic. Incomplete healing by the time a high school reunion or trip to St. Tropez rolls around can create anxiety. A fall in Google or Apple stock can interject a sense of guilt or regret. I always approach the patient's reaction with skepticism, knowing that it can change at the drop of a jowl.

The fact is people change. Their environments change. People react to change. People's reaction to change changes. And, to some, nothing may be as life-changing as plastic surgery.

With this in mind, when a patient asks how long any surgical result will last, after lecturing about technique and physiology and environmental factors, I ask them, "How long do you want it to last? How long did the face and body that God and nature originally give you last before you decided something needed 'fixing'?"

Patients may live with a perceived problem or deformity or imperfection for a variable length of time. When they claim to have been bothered by something for more than a few years, I ask them: Why now? If they were dissatisfied about their nose at sixteen, why are they doing a rhinoplasty at thirty-five? If they noted jowls ten years ago, why are they deciding to correct them now? If they had heavy, painful breasts for forty years, why did they wait so long to undergo breast reduction? The answers can be revealing and may indicate life changes.

"I finally saved enough money to have surgery."

"I lost (or am about to lose) my job and now I have to compete with all those young people."

"My wife/husband passed away last year and I am ready to look for another woman/man."

"I'm starting to look like my mother/grand-mother/older sister and I don't like it."

"The kids are out of the house and I want to do something for myself."

Just as people are tolerant of shortcomings for a variable length of time, they might live with a good or not-so-good surgical result for a variable length of time. While it is important to know how long a post-surgical result will stay comparably the same, it is not necessarily a predictor of emotional state or behavior, or surgical success. Some patients will jump in for a revision as soon as they detect some new or recurrent imperfection. Others will contently pass from this life old and withered with a torso or face riddled with "imperfections." Changes in one's life do not stop after plastic surgery.

In uncontrolled, flawed studies on the longevity of facelifts, it was found that the average interval between facelifts was about eight to twelve years.[5, 6] Thus was born the idea that a facelift lasts for seven to twelve years. While that quantitative "fact" sounds definitive, it is not. Imagine if you were someone who "had" to go in for a second surgery after three years. You might feel your surgeon wasn't very good because the first surgery didn't last. Or if it did "last" fifteen years, you'd think your surgeon was a genius. Of course, you'd have to say the same thing about God and your original face, depending on at what age you decided to undergo the operation in the first place! Why does one God-made face last for sixty years in one person, forty-five in another, and forever in most?

So, we cannot predict when, or even if, a person will decide to undergo a cosmetic procedure. We do not know how long a given result will persist. And we cannot portend when an individual will decide to have a second surgery. In the end, because cosmetic plastic surgery is unnecessary, the real answer to the question of how long the result will last is, **"It'll last as long as you, the patient, want it to last."** In fact, I have

5 Sundine, MJ, Kretsis, V, and Connell, BF, Longevity of SMAS Facial Rejuvenation and Support, *Plast. Reconstr Surg.* 2010 Jul;126(1):229-37.
6 Guyuron, B, Bohkari, F., Thomas, T.,Secondary rhytidectomy, *Plast Reconstr Surg.*, 1997;100:1281-1284.

had patients remove perfectly good breast implants because what they got in their twenties just didn't feel comfortable to them in their forties. One attractive, tall, blond woman with two young kids had me remove hers within a year since she unexpectedly felt out of place among the other more conservative and unenhanced suburban housewives. Recently, a patient of Greek descent who had a rhinoplasty as a young woman had an epiphany as a middle-aged mother and now wanted me to restore some of her ethnic features.

If we break down the process of having plastic surgery into its components, what really happens is happening on a daily, if not hourly, basis. We examine ourselves. We react to those things and people around us. People react to us. We formulate opinions and feelings about ourselves and we act, or don't act, to change ourselves. We go through this process when choosing what food to eat for breakfast, what clothes to wear in the morning, when to buy what car, when and why to change hairstyles, etc. etc. There isn't a formula. There isn't a rule. There isn't a law, except the permanence of impermanence.

The fact of the matter is that, despite the appearance to the contrary in environments like Beverly Hills, Las Vegas, and Rio de Janeiro, most people do not opt for cosmetic surgery, even though they desire it. Whatever face and body they possess ends up lasting them a lifetime. Each person has to individually determine when their face and/or body fail to outlast their own expectations and when a change in their face and/or body will produce a positive enough effect to justify the costs of plastic surgery.

Once they choose to avail themselves of the benefits of cosmetic surgery that same process of self-assessment that led them to their first procedure will determine if, and when, they will opt for a secondary procedure. Statistics, as hard or soft as they may be, are not particularly helpful to an individual. **Statistics are the *results* of individual behavior, not the determinants of it.** How long a surgery lasts is as much in the mind of the patient as it is in the hands of the surgeon.

CHAPTER 8:

ART AIN'T DONE 'TIL IT'S DONE

* * *

One of the most elusive and frustrating aspects of plastic surgery is the difficulty of predicting a surgical result. Given that cosmetic surgery is elective and not performed urgently, patients desire and seek precision and predictability. They expect this from their doctor. I know I would be looking for such reassurance if I were lying on an operating room table, staring at a masked face with a sharp, glistening scalpel in hand. In considering the concept of *cosmetic surgery as a creative endeavor,* having a clear idea of what one wants for an endpoint and then being able to communicate that endpoint between patient and surgeon is as important as being able to technically achieve it. Like much of life, as discussed by one of my mentors, Dr. D. Ralph Millard, Jr., in his book *The Principlization of Plastic Surgery,* you must have a goal. More importantly, the goal must be a common goal between patient and surgeon.

Plastic surgeons use photographs of celebrities and models to demonstrate an ideal goal. I analyze pictures of patients in their more youthful decades in order to see what changes have occurred, how they have occurred, and what I need to do to reset the clock. I sketch, draw, and explain anatomy and the changes that will hopefully produce the desired look. Some drawings are quite precise and some are merely schematic. Sometimes I measure angles. Often I will bring out a tape measure, ruler, or caliper. I might even use adhesive tape to temporarily modify a breast while discussing lifts and reductions. However I conjure up the image, the bottom line is that there must be a *meeting of the minds* between me and my patient. It is the crucial beginning of the artistic collaboration and it would be a potentially dangerous predicament for either of us to be unaware of the other's image.

Some patients are very intuitive and can understand surgical concepts without spending years going through medical school or surgical residency. Some can grasp the physical metamorphosis without the aid of a Frank Netter or DaVinci anatomical drawing. A few are artists themselves and will bring in professional renderings of their dreams complete with multiple views and three-dimensional shading. Most will ask to see before-and-after pictures. A number will even ask for, and expect, computerized representations of their final appearance. Not having such a concrete example of their wishes will discourage some from proceeding with surgery and may often drive these patients to other plastic surgeons who do use these technological capabilities. For better or worse, prospective patients do form judgments of surgeons based on these visual aids. They can be as invaluable selling points as they are planning tools.

It might seem self-serving to argue against the use of computerized morphing programs when I do not use one; I certainly could purchase one and learn how to manipulate screen images. With many technologies in medicine, if you have it, you will use it. In fact, one might feel compelled to exploit it at every chance and then it becomes its own raison d'être, a self-fulfilling necessity.

While morphing technologies can produce a lot of stunning and helpful images and may help us understand certain critical processes such as facial aging and post-surgical changes when used retrospectively, there is not an exact, prospective, predictable correlation between what one can do with a cursor and what one can do with a scalpel. In a study of rhinoplasty patients in 1998, actual post-surgical noses had 80 percent correlation with their respective pre-surgical computer-generated predictions: quite good, but not perfect. In fact, the 20 percent non-correlation is peculiarly similar to the accepted revision rate for primary rhinoplasty before the advent of computer imaging.[7] A more recent study in 2007 showed that 32 percent of computer-morphed images, as rated by experienced surgeons, did not realistically portray actual post-operative results.[8] This is not surprising since there are variables such as bleeding and swelling that differ between patients. Also, hard structure changes that

---

7 Among other, Punthakee, X., et al., Digital Imaging in Rhinoplasty, *Aesthetic Plastic Surgery*, Vol. 33(11) 635-638, 1998.
8 Patrocinio, L G., et al., Evaluation of Computer Imaging in Rhinoplasty: Patient's Satisfaction, *International Archives of Otorhinolaryngology*, Vol. 11(2), 2007.

can be reliably measured are not precisely mirrored in the accompanying soft tissue changes that comprise much of the surface contouring. The margin of error in surgery (and there is *always* a margin of error) is certainly greater than the precision of a computer-generated image. Surgical skills in the operating room are not the same as surgical concepts in one's head, although the latter might be a prerequisite for the former. Finally, surgical techniques are not consistently reproducible between surgeons, as much as computerized manipulations are. That is, surgical maneuvers are *less* predictable than computer-generated maneuvers especially when operating on soft tissues.

Another finding in this study was even more disappointing; the rating surgeons felt the post-operative results were actually *worse* than the morphed images twenty-five percent of the time.

The computer certainly enhances the communication process between doctor and patient, but may add another variable that the patient must judge (i.e., the computer skills of the surgeon). A surgeon could actually be better at computers or drawing, for that matter, than at surgery. Furthermore, in some practices, the morphing is not even performed by the operating surgeon but by surgical consultants. That seems to be an obvious disconnect.

Another potential problem beside the patient not being told of, or not grasping, the inaccuracy of the technology is that there is an implied, or presumed, precision *promised* by computers and their software that may not be surgically *reproducible*. When prospective patients are shown possible results on a computer, even though warned by a written disclaimer against truly expecting these results, there is an inevitable imprinting of these images that is difficult to ignore, compounded by the patient's own wishful thinking. How literally a person takes the computer-generated image can be the difference between a happy patient and a disappointed one.

Asking a person to discount a visual image may be more difficult than forgetting a verbal one. It may be similar to asking a jury to disregard an inappropriate testimony or piece of evidence; it is hard to stuff the genie back into the bottle. Imagine if Judge Ito had asked the jury to try to ignore Johnny Cochrane's "If it doesn't fit, you must acquit" glove demonstration at O.J. Simpson's murder trial.

The computer may indeed be helpful, but not infallible, as one might expect. Leading medical liability insurers, such as the Doctor's Company, also echo a caveat regarding implied results of computer imaging, stressing that the images can help in screening unrealistic expectations but may not represent actual results. The complexities of technique, the variation in anatomy, and, especially, the vicissitudes of what is desired may all impact the before-and-after photos. One might justifiably ask, "If it isn't accurate, why show it at all?"

For me, it is helpful to put plastic surgery within the construct of an artistic and creative, not strictly scientific, endeavor—which it truly is. It is more like performance art than structural art. And it is certainly more like original art than reproduction art, even though we strive to make our surgical techniques predictable and reproducible for every patient.

One fundamental contradiction is that a surgeon should be able to show that he has performed a certain procedure before, yet plastic surgeons are always inventing, reinventing, and creating variations on surgical techniques. Cosmetic surgery is a *constantly* evolving field. In fact, it might be said that a surgeon who mechanically performs the same procedure, or same sequence of technical maneuvers, on every patient is not doing the patient justice. This is especially true of rhinoplasty, where traditional reduction rhinoplasty (i.e., making a large nose smaller) was a series of identical steps producing a distinctive, telltale, and identifiable post-operative result that is now being replaced with a more fluid, flexible, and customized paradigm. The same is true of breast reduction and breast lifts, where adherence to a predetermined, reproducible, and mathematical pattern results in very similar end results. Again this approach is being supplanted by a more individualized and varied end result depending on patient desire.

Any artist goes through a preparatory phase visualizing the end result, whether it is a stage play, a musical performance, or an athletic sequence. There is a subset of science and psychology devoted to the imagery that we are taught as children. "Hit the ball, Johnny. You can do it!" "Visualize your hand going through the bricks." "You think, therefore you are."

Preparation means there is "practice, practice, and more practice." There are rehearsals. An artist may produce sketches or models. A performer might play words, music, or actions over and over again in his mind. Visualization is extremely important to many artists, including me. I will rehearse an operation many times over in my mind prior to the actual surgery like preparing for a violin recital, even dreaming about it while I sleep or thinking about it when I exercise. I anticipate various scenarios and play out multiple options so that I am as prepared as I can be when I finally sit down to perform the real surgery in front of the anesthetized patient. For that one performance, and one particular audience, for which a patient has expended much time, money, and effort, I, the surgeon as artist, do what I hope to do in the manner and with the results that I intend. I can do all the preparations I want. But in the end, **art ain't done til it's actually done.**

All the photographs, sketches, descriptions, drawings, and analysis come down to the few minutes or hours in the operating room performing the art. You have to be prepared, but it is still art and subject to the vicissitudes of the moment. "Hope for the best and plan for the worst." It is what happens in real life, in firefighting, in real estate investing, in the kitchen, in the operating room, on the tennis court or baseball field, and in any creative endeavor. As much as we would like to, and as much as patients demand it, we cannot always predict what will happen as we perform. The ability to adapt to the moment may be the difference between success and failure.

It is extremely important to communicate to patients what uncertainties exist in plastic surgery. Nothing in plastic surgery is a hundred percent. In our rush to get patients on the operating room table, and recognizing the practical realities of cosmetic surgery as less of a branch of medicine and more of a consumer-driven business, plastic surgeons, or more often their assistants, may describe the proposed transformation in gilded verbal shorthand.

"It's a piece of cake."

"You're going to look fabulous."

"I've done this a thousand times before."

"Your face will be perfect."

All of this may be true and ninety-nine times out of one hundred (even nine hundred and ninety-nine out of a thousand) things may go without a hitch. We all need confidence and reassurances. No one likes negativity; the partner to positive imagery is the *absence of negativity.* But this still does not mean that an expectation will be achieved and be satisfactory to the patient.

Looking at plastic surgery as art is not intended to be pessimistic. You don't stop going to the theater because an actor may possibly forget his or her lines. You don't stop going to the symphony because of the uncertainty of knowing how Beethoven's Fifth is going to be played this time around. You don't stop going to a ballgame because your home team might lose or stop watching the ballplayers try to hit .300 because you know they will fail to hit safely 70 percent of the time. You go because there is an expectation that you will be entertained in a positive way and that your quality of life will be enhanced. There is a fine line between having too much expectation so that you are easily dissatisfied and having such tempered expectation that you are not disappointed by shortcomings or prevented from wanting success. Thankfully, most audiences have *reasonable* expectations. This is also what makes a good plastic surgical candidate.

Accepting plastic surgery as art, *unnecessary but desirable* art, allows patients to understand it in a more realistic way and will force them to look at themselves in a more honest manner. One has to accept that there are nuances, imperfections, and unpredictability in cosmetic surgery. Perceived problems and final performances are subject to interpretation. That's why it's important to go with experienced performers.

Because art is pliable, it requires patients to be accountable to their own selves. Rather than simply lying down for the surgeon like diners blindly awaiting a chef's choice, patients must take an active role in the artistic process. They become collaborators with the surgeon, commissioners of a work of art. They will become the artist, with the surgeon forming the hands and consciousness of the artist. How the art is attained is as much a function of the patient as it is of the surgeon.

Almost every artist will have his or her portfolio or sample of the past work. Looking at a surgeon's brag book, a photo album or, more likely these days, a DVD is invariably part of the consultation. While I never refuse to show patients pictures of other patients, I am not convinced that the reasons the photos are being shown are clear or that they are received in the way they are intended.

Most articles giving advice to prospective patients tell them to ask the surgeon to show before-and-after photos. Even our professional society has a picture gallery of surgical results. One reason is to assure the patient that the surgeon has done a certain type, number, or variety of procedures. If a surgeon has no photos to show, that can give a patient an uneasy feeling. However, as indicated previously, not having done a procedure before doesn't necessarily mean it is not the appropriate thing to do or that the surgeon is not going to do a good job. If you think of all the great artists in their respective fields, they invariably excelled in many different areas. Mozart composed minuets, concertos, quartets, operas, and symphonies. Picasso painted, sketched, sculpted, and did set designs. Shakespeare wrote sonnets, tragedies, and comedies.

Michelangelo created drawings, murals, architecture, and sculptures. Innovation, versatility, and adaptability are hallmarks of great artistic minds.

Another reason one looks at photos is that hopefully you will see similar patients with similar procedures getting similar results. Unfortunately, this is rarely, if ever, the case. In fact, the official website of our national society, while displaying photos of actual patients, gives a disclaimer that discounts the applicability of the end results to specific individual patients. Not only is this a necessary legal statement, but it is also the truth. So how useful can these photos be?

Obviously, the problem is that most patients are not looking at photos in order to be screened in or out as candidates. They are looking for results they can identify with within their goals and expectations and, in the process, consciously or subconsciously, they are forming judgments about that surgeon.

Brag books usually have an array of patients with many dissimilar features. Similarities apparent to a layperson may ignore dissimilarities evident only to a plastic surgeon. For example, the correction to a patient's sagging neck may miss the disparities in a patient's cheekbone or mandible or amount of fat, which have great influence on the type and effectiveness of any facial "lift." Loose skin just under the chin is not the same as loose skin further down on the neck. But they all look the same to the layperson. A patient's breasts may look the same size but her chest may have a different width or curvature that will affect the way identical implants influence those breasts. Liposuction on the abdomen may not take into account the tone of the unseen underlying muscles that may be more influential than the fat or skin in producing a given contour.

Even if you were to find a complete match, that does not have any predictability about future cases. As I tell patients, doing plastic surgery is not like buying a Sony television.

I will caution patients that while photographs are necessary to the process of evaluation, they are also limited in their value. They provide only a static two-dimensional view that does not demonstrate or evaluate the three-dimensional structure, nor the effect of the fourth dimension of time. For example, while I take pictures of the abdomen and neck flexed as well as when the patient is fully erect, surgery cannot control or eliminate the looseness or folding that occurs. This is mainly due to the elasticity or quality of the soft tissues that cannot be captured in photographs. The effects of motion are not directly addressed by surgery except by what can be affected by manipulation of muscles. Many patients are concerned about their appearance in non-standard pose positions or when moving, such as the excess bulging that they see in their abdomen when sitting or the wrinkles in their face while talking or animating. The patient will learn and need to accept the limitations their surgery will have on these *dynamic* qualities.

One might get a sense about the surgeon by looking at post-surgical results. Sometimes all the noses look similar. Sometimes all the breast augmentations have the same general shape or size. I get that comment all the time. "I went to such and such doctor, and all his faces look like this or all his noses look like that." However, then you have to know whether this is a function of the surgeon or his patient population. The paternalistic surgeon might decide that all patients look best with a particular characteristic, such as high-arched brows or pointed noses or square jaws. If you like that look, you're in luck. If you don't like that look, you might want to try another doctor.

But what if the doctor is not a paternalistic doctor and is just doing what the patient wants? Then you might be making a mistake by presuming he is not the surgeon for you. You might not like the results but all the patients might be happy patients. And what if you like what you see but your particular anatomy does not lend itself to an identical result? What if you don't see anything that resembles your anatomy or anything that you like? Does that mean you are out of luck?

There might even be more value in seeing photos where all the patients are indeed different with different results. That might mean that the surgeon is more versatile, more differential in his or her thinking, more "artistic," if you will.

So what is the answer with patient photos? The most that before-and-after photos can do is perhaps allow the patient to expose what *she* thinks. By commenting on what she sees in the photos, she reveals parts of herself: what she likes or doesn't like, what she finds attractive or offensive. She cannot, however, make accurate judgments about the surgeon's skill. She is, in fact, revealing more about herself as a discerning subject than the photos are revealing about the surgeon as a skillful artist. Of course, this is not the usual patient's intent when she asks to look at photos. She is looking for something about the surgeon and his skill or judgment, so there may be a *disconnect* between what the photos show and what the patients *want* the photos to show. Often a patient will compare photos of one surgeon with those from another to help her choose between surgeons. I am not convinced that this auditioning process is a valid approach, but it is what happens.

I explain to my patients that every patient that sits in my easy chair is like a blank canvas. Without their input, I do not know what to put on the canvas. I do not make presumptions about what they want to hang over their bed or display on their living room mantle. The more information they can give me about what pleases them, the closer I can get towards making them satisfied. Often showing me what they don't want to look like is more informative and important than showing what they do want. Or, as I put it, if they want to get to the Waldorf Astoria in New York City from Los Angeles and they hate the Marriott and Miami, I might not be able to get them a specific room at the Waldorf, but I sure don't want them to end up in the Marriott in Miami (no offense to the Marriott or Miami).

If they see a result they don't like, whether in before-and-after photos or the lay-media, it might be possible to avoid that type of look or it can be used as a focal point to discuss some aspect of a procedure, such as a particular complication or side effect that can occur. In fact, some plastic surgeons use other plastic surgeons' before-and-after photos just to demonstrate possible surgical outcomes. And some brag books will only have results the surgeon believes give him those bragging rights. Results that do not pass muster do not get put in front of the patient; the patient cannot judge that which she doesn't see.

Perhaps photos are like an artist's résumé showing the artist's experience, style and, hopefully, competence. But it may not be completely predictive of the next work of art. It is much more valuable when viewed with the editorial comments of the actual surgeon and not a surgical consultant or nurse unfamiliar with the nuances of the work, and only after getting to know the surgeon personally to see where the surgeon is coming from.

By themselves, without editorial comments, photos are not very helpful. What may be more helpful is to know how former patients felt about their experience and individual results regardless of what the actually results are. Did the surgeon give the patient what he or she wanted? Was it a pleasant process? Was the surgeon responsive to their desires and honest in his assessment? What a patient actually looks like is less important than whether or not they are satisfied with the results. **Before-and-after photos do not reveal patient satisfaction.**

So what is a prospective patient to do with this?

The difficulty a patient faces is the same difficulty and challenge a plastic surgeon faces. How to make a decision in the face of uncertainty? That is why there is something to be said about a patient's maturity. It is why a doctor's experience is important. It is why artists must practice their craft. We must somehow reconcile our need and desire for predictability with the intrinsic presence of uncertainty in an artistic endeavor. It is why medicine, and especially plastic surgery, is an art and not merely a science. Science implies certainty and predictability, although even then we have the *Heisenberg Uncertainty Principle* and *Einstein's Theory of Relativity.* Surgery is based on science but is not exactly scientific. This seems quite obvious after a bit of contemplation but is a challenge to accept when lying on your back, facing a knife held by your surgeon whose face is hidden by a mask.

The most important step in creating a work of art is to have a goal or a purpose and then make that first step in perhaps a series of steps of collaborative planning. Any art has a **creator**, such as the composer, a **facilitator** or **artist**, such as the musician or painter or actor, the **medium**, such as acrylic or clay or the spoken or sung word, and an **audience**, whether of one or of a million. In great art, all four components interact and are interdependent. In plastic surgery, the interesting thing is that all of the components of the art should include the patient. The patient should be a creative partner. Certainly the patient and her anatomy is the medium. She can help or hurt the facilitating artist-surgeon by being cooperative or being noncompliant. She is also the most important audience and, in fact for me, the only audience that matters. The patient, *not* the surgeon, is the focal point of my art.

In many ways, plastic surgery is a paradigm for life. The "art of life" or the "art of living" are catch phrases that have often been used as a rallying cry or slogan. **"Plastic Surgery as Art"** is the motto for my medical practice. What it implies, what it requires, and what I tell my patients is that you can practice the art, and plan, draw, and rehearse the art, and talk and consult about the art. And that is all necessary. But in the end, when standing or sitting, or lying down, face-to-face, on the operating room table, there is a process that must occur and that is, for some, like a religious experience. It involves a "leap of faith" and trust based on knowledge. And it occurs both for a patient as well as for the surgeon—just like having faith in science or trusting your golf swing. Once you take that leap, a self-confident calm appears that gives predictability and future outcome a fighting chance. And that is all we can hope for in the first place…a reasonable chance of success.

Directors tell actors to trust their instincts. Coaches must trust their players' abilities. Artists must trust their feelings, and musicians must trust their technique. Parents learn to trust their children's decisions. Spouses must trust each other to be secure in a mature relationship. Trust must substitute for absolute predictability in the operating room. The patients must have it and the surgeon must have it. More than showing patients photographs, I will offer patients the opportunity and the right to talk to other patients. It is an effective way of building trust in a surgeon. The visual end result shown in brag books is not nearly as important as the satisfaction of the actual patient. In an extreme example, I tell my patients that it matters not what the singer Michael Jackson looked like, but only what he himself thought about what he looked like; so, too, of more common patients. The proof is not in the picture. The proof is in the approval. If they are happy, then I am happy, as long as they are safe.

Once the all-important trust is obtained—and it is a mutual trust—the art can begin. The patient relinquishes his or her body to the surgeon's knife and the surgeon then begins the technical application that, like musical technique, will determine if the art has a chance of being successful. Technique is necessary, but insufficient, to guarantee a positive outcome. It is only after the completion of all the meticulous, honest, soul-searching and artistic preliminary planning that trust is put to the test and that the surgeon's skill will attempt to make the image become the art…because **art ain't done 'til it's done.**

CHAPTER 9:

THE GUILT OF THE V-WORD

* * *

Sitting across from her, I can tell she is nervous. Words come hesitantly. Her eyes look away as I fix my gaze on her face. She plays with the rings on her fingers. Although fully clothed, it is as if she is completely disrobed and vulnerable for the first time in her life. She is a quiet woman with a couple of grown kids and a well-paying job. She has a hint of crinkles around the eyes and a touch of maternal gray in her hair.

"I know it's such an insignificant thing," she says defensively.

"Everything's relative," I reply with gentle reassurance.

"I've got two kids," she seems to confess.

"Congratulations."

"I love my job," she declares with some force, as if trying to convince me.

"So do I."

"My husband adores me," she states, afraid that I might think differently and assume that an absence of attention is why she is in my office.

"That's even better."

But that isn't why she is here. She is searching for the right phrase to express herself. I just sit and wait because truth often comes from silence, like prayer or meditation, or, as we said in college, just contemplating your navel. Then it comes.

"It's vanity," she confesses. "Just vanity."

There it is: the V-word.

The V-word seems to admit self-absorption, superficiality, selfishness, and narcissism. It hints at turmoil beneath the skin surface. It suggests a vacuum in the soul. It implies having no value—at least no lasting value. By definition, it refers to an *excessive* concern for, or pride in, one's appearance. There seems to be nothing good about the V-word except that admitting it can be self-revealing and possibly life-changing. Most whisper the word as if it is an apology. Some claim it unapologetically as if they deserve the forbidden treasures proscribed by society except by way of the V-word. "Yes," some might proclaim. "I'm vain and proud of it." Not her. She says it in a whisper. But it is there for both of us to hear.

Her sense of guilt when the V-word comes out is palpable. I almost expect her to bolt from the chair and run to her room like a schoolchild embarrassed after admitting a terrible misdeed. But she doesn't. She says it like it is part of her and she is ready, willing, and able to take her punishment as if atoning for her sin. I sense a breakthrough, a lifting of a veil.

"It's just these bags and these wrinkles. My body's not perfect, but it's okay. It doesn't bother me. But I can't stand looking tired. I don't feel old, but I look old. It's kind of ridiculous...looking younger. I'm just being vain." There, in fifteen seconds, is what she fears, what she feels, what she likes, and what she wants.

She is a mature woman: educated, possibly with an advanced degree, articulate, knowledgeable, contemplative, forthcoming. She is a professional woman with teenage kids and a husband who loves her. She is concerned about her kids. She worries about their studies and about their future. She is loyal to her husband, loves his strengths, and laughs at his foibles. She reads about war, gas prices, and natural disasters. She knows the world has to find an answer to AIDS, poverty, child abuse, and terrorism. She shops for bargains, frequents a place of worship regularly, and loves to travel to new places. But here she is talking about bags and wrinkles.

It does seem so disproportionate and incongruous, even belittling to one's pride. How do you compare fat with cancer, jowls with global warming, and sagging breasts with corporate bankruptcies and fraud? How can you not be apologetic for worrying about fine lines when young men are dying overseas and in inner cities? More importantly, how do I, as custodian and facilitator of such "vain" expression, reconcile my very own existence and purpose in the milieu of universal, and seemingly more important, issues?

One of my medical school classmates and former roommate is a world-renowned AIDS researcher and a *Time Magazine* "Man of the Year." Another classmate was a U.S. senator and former prospective presidential candidate. Others are doing significant research or running major institutions and medical departments in prestigious hospitals. Another friend is the world's most beloved cellist and yet another childhood friend a celebrated female CEO of a Fortune 500 company employing forty thousand people. The V-word does seem so imposing in its insignificance and self-interest. Right behind follows guilt in its shadow. I am bonded to this patient by the V-word and its implications. I might not be saving the world, but what I do and say is important to her.

I can ignore the V-word and proceed on my merry way. I can walk this road with her towards the operating room in silent complicity: the two of us like a couple not willing or able to face the extramarital affair that both know exists or the divisive argument we just had the night before about some extraneous and expensive purchase. I could laugh it off or say something smart and flippant like, "Oh, aren't we all a bit vain?" or "Well, I hope you are vain because otherwise there would be no reason for you to be here!" Ha, ha, ha... The problem is that ignoring her feelings of vanity is also ignoring the vein of guilt lurking beneath the surface that threatens to undermine a patient's commitment and self-confidence.

Obviously there is a spectrum of guilt an individual might feel. One can be completely devoid of guilt (as in psychopathic or selfish individuals who don't give a hoot about others). On the other hand, guilt can be an extreme burden (as in those paralyzed by self-critique and self-flagellation). Yet all patients who unapologetically embrace cosmetic surgery are not sociopathic—hardly—and all patients who are racked with guilt (and subsequently reject potentially life-changing surgery) are not self-sacrificing or self-righteous. One can just as easily praise the former as an unabashed, self-improving role model while criticize the latter as an old-fashioned and unenlightened self-defeatist. We all have varying degrees of narcissism—some healthy, some very destructive—and varying degrees of self-doubt. And that certainly includes doctors, especially plastic surgeons.

The guilt associated with the V-word begs the question: What is important? Of course, that depends on who you are. You will never feel guilty fighting for the things you believe are important. Everyone, every group, every nation has its own individual concerns. You won't feel guilty standing up for your children, defending your family, or feeding the poor. However, trouble starts when you lose conviction in what you believe in or when a person you respect or care about, perhaps even yourself, criticizes or harshly judges your actions or beliefs. Children can't understand why mothers need to be so clean, so a mother may begin to feel guilty when her cleanliness affects the way the children act. Husbands can't understand why wives need to have so many shoes, so the wives might feel guilty when the husband they love protests. Wives can't understand why husbands have to have so many tools, so the husband may sense guilt when the wife he cares so much about complains. You are free from guilt when you are *not* aligned with those expressing disapproval. People do not have to be aligned with everyone. Muslims are not aligned with Christians. Socialists reject capitalism. Pacifists don't back the NRA. None of these groups will feel much guilt about their beliefs in the face of their counterpart's critique.

In America, the Declaration of Independence, among other guarantees, asserts the right of all citizens to "Life, Liberty, and the *Pursuit of Happiness.*" This right is not dependent on anyone else's approval. Doesn't that pretty much cover getting rid of bags and wrinkles, love handles, sagging breasts, and whatever else bothers you? Who is to judge what an individual considers important to his or her state of happiness? There does not appear to be need for apologies, self-doubt, or sense of guilt if you are a citizen of the United States of America. Even Benjamin Franklin said that while you have the right to the pursuit of happiness, "you still have to catch it yourself." Vanity seems constitutionally protected, even encouraged.

One of my friends has dozens, perhaps hundreds, of designer T-shirts in her bedroom drawer (readers can substitute their own personal experiences with tools, shoes, toys, and golf clubs), most of which she has never worn. Yet she loves to shop for additional T-shirts, many of which she will never wear or let see the light of day out of that drawer. While I might want her to feel a little guilty (which she doesn't), or perhaps a bit silly (which she might), about this apparently enjoyable, but seemingly purposeless, pastime, it, on reflection, is akin to her trying to make me feel guilty about spending a hundred dollars and five hours trying to put a little white ball into eighteen tiny cups in the middle of a desert—every week and sometimes twice a week. It would be futile because I know I wouldn't feel guilty playing golf, unless I were doing it during the birth of my children—which I wasn't. We each have a vested self-interest in our own activities, but not necessarily in those of the other. Her shopping doesn't impact my life and my poor putting doesn't offend hers. If we are ever aligned, guilt might set in. So guilt requires wavering of conviction and disapproval by someone you care about or respect, and whose life you affect.

The opposite of the conflict between self-interest and non-self-interest is a compassionate and unifying acceptance of others. That is, when the concerns and interests of an individual coincide with those of others, be it a partner, a family, a culture, or a nation, then guilt disappears. Guilt requires some form of disapproval or disharmony. The cause or the idea or the feeling is validated and becomes guilt-free by its common denominator; there is a meeting of the minds. If I love shopping for designer T-shirts then everyone is happy. The husband enjoys watching his wife shop for shoes. The wife takes pride in the tinkering the husband does in the garage. The child loves the fact that everything and everyone at home looks and smells so clean. Oh, well, maybe not that.

In my encounter with patients, reconciliation can be the meeting of the two minds within a single patient: the vanity mind and the guilt-laden mind. Or, it can be the mind of a patient meeting the mind of whoever is around judging her. That is what I am after when consulting with a patient: a meeting of the minds. Until that time, vanity and guilt do battle. "Should I or shouldn't I?" "It's okay, it's not okay." "I want it. I don't need it."

Vanity and guilt are influential in the beauty and plastic surgery industry. They both polarize beliefs and actions, and can motivate or paralyze individuals. If patients were completely devoid of elements of vanity, cosmetic surgeons would have no patients. There has to be some concern for one's appearance: That's the business we are in. Every patient who comes in for consultation is, in his or her own way, balancing vanity and guilt. I am ever vigilant about how a patient interprets and accepts, or rejects, each since it may critically impact the success or failure of surgery.

Some make no apologies for their vanity and thus enter surgery guilt-free. Then it is incumbent on me to measure the reasonableness of the patient's decision to have surgery since the patient may not have his or her own internal checks and balances. These are the patients who plow single-mindedly and without constraints toward improving or changing their appearance to the exclusion of everything else: the Barbie doll syndrome. They are consumed by appearance and not at all racked by guilt. They are the train wreck that is delayed by each subsequent procedure.

Others, however, will feel guilty for what they are doing right up to the moment they are put to sleep. That last-minute doubt can sow the seeds of regret if things are not as perfect as they desire. They are the train wreck that might happen should anything not go according to plan.

When a patient directly mentions or alludes to the V-word, visions of Narcissus, or perhaps even Icarus, come to mind. One can go from simply looking at oneself or needing to escape some imprisonment to wanting to go beyond mere earthly existence and soar towards the sun, not listening to the voice of reason, safety, and moderation Beginning from a simple act of self-examination or desire for self-improvement comes a life of self-destruction and unhappiness; this is not entirely unheard of in cosmetic surgery. This can range from an unrelenting pursuit of perfection to persistent dissatisfaction with inherent imperfection. Neither situation is healthy or happy. Plastic surgeons are, or should be, constantly on the lookout for the destructive self-hate and obsessive self-love (or lack thereof) masquerading as the desire for self-improvement.

There are an infinite number of psychological reasons for patients to seek cosmetic alteration. Because of the possible inner turmoil and secret motivations, plastic surgeons must, but don't always, look beyond the physical imperfections and examine the patient for elements of vanity and guilt. We must then judge their balance.

On the other side of the surgical table, plastic surgeons may struggle themselves with the feeling of guilt for operating on "easy" targets (i.e., the patient who appears motivated but is really psycho-emotionally vulnerable). We may want to save these patients from themselves by refusing surgery, referring them to psychiatrists, or, conversely, trying improbably to make them happy by justifying surgery because "if not me, then someone less qualified." Some of us really do struggle with our personal beliefs in whether or not to commit to surgery because there is no specific test or dark line that a patient, or plastic surgeon, can cross that delineates a good candidate from a bad. There are areas of gray. The fact is there are degrees and gray areas of sociopath behavior and narcissistic personalities. What patients may rightly feel guilty about is not necessarily vanity but a simple desire for self-improvement based on healthy self-love.

Wanting to have a shapelier breast or a more attractive nose or a less unhappy or tired look is not vanity, just as wanting to wear flattering makeup or dress in nice clothes or drive a stylish car is not necessarily vanity. There is nothing wrong with wanting to look and feel your best. Let me repeat: **There is nothing wrong**

with wanting to look and feel your best! This is not only a human characteristic but also one found readily and widely in the entire animal kingdom.

The practice of physically altering the body is not a curse of Western civilization or first-world, developed countries. Pride in a beautiful place one can call "home" is universal. Think of how you feel when a person enters your home and says, "What a beautiful home you have." Our body is our home. Adornment of the face is as common in aboriginal cultures as it is in twenty-first century America. Scarification of the body as a form of cosmetic enhancement in African tribes has been around longer than silicone gel breast implants or laser face peels. Binding of feet in China, molding the skull in Egypt, and elongating the neck in Thailand were all taking place centuries before Columbus discovered America.

It is not a weakness to want to look attractive. There is absolutely nothing wrong with wanting to impress or gain favor with the opposite (or even the same) gender. Primping and preening have long-standing evolutionary roots in the animal kingdom and are distinctly tied to the survival and propagation of a species. Using physical beauty and enhancing it to bolster one's ego and confidence and to compete for the attention of a potential partner is basic to the preservation of lineage, whether individual or a species. In blunt and stark terms, if you don't attract, your lineage, or even your species, dies.

On the other hand, if a woman *doesn't* pay attention to the way she looks, some might presume that that woman has no pride in herself or is, God forbid, asexual. The same might be said of a man. Being disheveled and unconcerned with one's physique might earn the man a reputation of being unkempt, a slob, slovenly, or, again, having no pride in himself. No one would intentionally wish for such a reputation. Apologies for maintaining attractiveness are unnecessary.

Of course, no self-respecting plastic surgeon would *automatically* dismiss a person (who claims to be apologetic about showing concern for a physical imperfection) because they seem *too* guilt-laden. After all, these are exactly the people for whom cosmetic surgery is intended. Who wants to operate on perfect people with no claims of imperfection or who have no awareness or sensitivity to their perceived deformity? Aren't the vain the reason for cosmetic surgery's very existence? Without a person's concern for his or her external appearance, cosmetic surgery, as well as the entire beauty and fashion industry, would be unnecessary and extinct. Claiming sheepishly to be vain just highlights the introspection and sensitivity the patient is experiencing and underscores the patient's understanding of the seriousness of cosmetic surgery.

Concern for a perceived imperfection or deformity can be healthy or unhealthy; where that transition occurs is not well-defined or universally apparent to everyone. Traditional and conventional wisdom within the plastic surgical community holds that the more inverse the relationship between the concern for a deformity and the actual magnitude of the deformity, the less healthy is that concern. For example, if a patient is socially paralyzed by a small nasal bump or a minor facial wrinkle, a plastic surgeon might conclude that cosmetic surgery is inappropriate and that the patient is a high risk for being dissatisfied because of some underlying personality disorder, insecurity, or inferiority complex. At the opposite end of the spectrum, one might conclude that such a patient is, in fact, a good surgical risk since the correction or elimination of the anatomical problem is relatively simple.

We all have witnessed stories of how a simple operation can turn a patient's life around. In fact, that is what we relish. Who wouldn't want to turn a reclusive duck into a self-confident swan with one swipe of a scalpel or a few quick turns with a nasal rasp? Anytime we make a significant impact in the quality of a person's life by applying the tricks and tools of our trade, we feel that our education was worth it. Why? Because besides the improvement in that individual's quality of life, we know that happy people are likely to be more productive and less destructive to society than unhappy ones. That's the bigger picture.

So, then, how do we measure vanity? When does the concern for one's appearance and concern for one's self and our quality of life become a reflection of a bottomless pit of destructive self-love and self-hate? When are these concerns more an amplified distortion of reality? What does a plastic surgeon say when a potential patient apologizes for her (or his) vanity? Is she begging for a surgical cure, hinting at a non-surgical treatment, fishing for a reassuring editorial comment, or inviting someone to help enable the narcissism? What are we surgeons to do with all that guilt?

Vanity is a matter of degree and priorities. Balance is the key to the V-word. Combing one's hair can be a simple act of good grooming if done for five or ten seconds or a pathological manifestation of vanity if done for hours on end. Wanting to remove signs of aging can go hand-in-hand with a zest for life if one can accept *some* signs of aging, or it can be an expression of obsessive-compulsive disorder if the patient cannot tolerate *any* wrinkles or sagging. Wanting cosmetic surgery that will not prolong life but can increase enjoyment of life can be uplifting to the soul if one already enjoys life. Or, it can be an unfortunate proof of vanity—or, even worse, body dysmorphic disorder—if one forsakes the necessary and important things of life like education, food, housing, family, and social interaction.

Plastic surgeons should be wary of operating on people with body dysmorphic disorder (also referred to as imagined ugliness syndrome), since these patients tend to be consistently dissatisfied with the results of surgery. They have a psychological, not a physical or anatomical, disorder or defect. Reportedly affecting 1 to 2 percent of the population, this disorder goes beyond normal concerns with appearance and grooming, and beyond even the "vanity" that motivates many so-called plastic surgery junkies. People with BDD lack adequate insight and may frankly be delusional.

Patients who are driven by vanity want to obtain a certain perfection or attractiveness or beauty that is not necessarily unthinkable or unobtainable, but is prioritized inappropriately or have goals that can never be realized. They may not see anything wrong with their appearance but may be blinded by the need to improve or better their self physically.

Patients with body dysmorphic disorder do not see themselves as normal and do not necessarily want to be attractive or beautiful. Rather, they are driven by a *mis*perception of what they look like and a desire to blend in or appear normal; this is impossible because of their skewed interpretation of who they are. Most patients have a *healthy* concern with appearance and will not let it control their lives or distort their perception of who they are. They are not vain. Their desire for self-improvement is not cloaked in self-destruction or misplaced priorities. However, there is always a possibility that, in the aftermath of an unexpected complication, this healthy path of self-improvement may inadvertently detour onto an unhealthy path of self-destruction.

Each patient has her own motivation and personal view of her appearance and world. I believe it is appro- priate and helpful, if not critically important, to reas- sure her that her healthy and reasonable search for a plastic surgical solution to her anatomic concern is indeed healthy and reasonable. It is important that her sense of vanity is not a form of self-destructive van- ity that will compromise her ability to be content.

A disproportionate emoting of guilt associated with a confession of presumed vanity is not helpful. It can affect a rational analysis of the anatomic problem. It may compound the anxiety and interfere with the ability to make a decision when a complication, unac- ceptable result, or catastrophe occurs. Clear thought is as important as a steady hand. Being able to redefine vanity to the patient and convince her with an objec- tive analysis of her anatomy that she is reasonable in concern and expectation is part of the preoperative preparation. In the end, assuaging her guilt in want- ing to undertake the surgery is a big step towards per- forming the correct procedure. All this sets the stage for a positive response. Of course, if her actions are truly vain, as evidenced by a disproportionate concern with an imperceptible deformity or her neglect of home, family, and necessities of life, then I will bring her attention to that.

The guilt of vanity is a negative feeling that places my patient at odds with herself from the outset and fosters a potential for regret that can only produce elements of unhappiness and dissatisfaction. As a trip to the operating room is like a trip down the aisle, where self-defeating, self-doubting, and self-critical thoughts can be emotionally disastrous; both of us will want to be as certain as we can be about the reasons we are taking this journey. Anything I can do to define or redefine the V-word, put it in perspective, and place guilt to rest is going to add to a positive attitude and successful experience for my patient.

CHAPTER 10:

PLASTIC SURGERY IS WORTH A THOUSAND WORDS

Fabulous, rejuvenate, youthful, sculpted, enhance,
subtle, settle, fantastic, beautify, augment,
unnatural, voluptuous,
better, extraordinary, younger, weird,
over-done, excessive, plump,
proportional, restore, replenish, natural,
perky, elegant, artistic, exotic,
renew, shapely, terrific, curvaceous,
incredible, anti-aging,
fountain of youth, contouring, gorgeous,
lift, tighten, tweak,
nip, tuck, exaggerate, sensual, improve,
perfect, reduce,
attractive, soften, smooth, gentle, harmonize...

* * *

There is a host of words commonly heard in cosmetic surgery conversations over prosciutto,
mozzarella. and tomato salad or during private consultations in well-appointed medical offices. As in John
Baldessari's work *Terms Most Useful in Describing Creative
Works of Art* (1966-1968), most of these words are emotional, qualitative, or descriptive in nature and are

not absolute, quantitative, or measurable. We use and accept the above terms so easily, yet they are often the least practical for plastic surgeons. We need more than their imagined implications. More importantly, we require precise, analytical, and anatomic definitions.

Beauty is a subjective term. While tossed about so nonchalantly like some off-handed greeting, beauty, like its definition, is illusive. It comes in many shapes and sizes. When seeking beauty, a patient often won't, or can't, define exactly what needs to be done or what specific goals need to be met. It is not like batting .300, rushing one hundred yards per game, or acing a tennis ball at one hundred and thirty miles per hour. Those goals can be measured and judged without argument. You either achieve your goal or not. Beauty is as ephemeral and mysterious as it is obvious. Men know a "10" when they see her, but each person's standards may be different.

Plastic surgeons have to translate "beauty" or "youthful" or "elegant" into anatomic terms. Like pornography, beauty is hard to define but one often thinks he knows it when he sees it. But this is not always true. Stereotypical Eastern beauty is different from stereotypical Western beauty. Eastern interpretation of Western beauty is different from Western interpretation of Western beauty. What is not beautiful in one society (e.g., keloids in Beverly Hills) may be a symbol of beauty in another (e.g., scarification patterns in Baule people of the Ivory Coast). Beauty in youth (e.g., the low-lying brows of teenage models) is not beauty in middle age (e.g., when brows are lifted). We talk about cultural, or ethnic, beauty: African beauty, Asian beauty, Romanesque beauty, Southern beauty, aging beauty, classic beauty. The multitude of ways the word is used should clue us in to the variability of the word. And what are the quantitative differences between *beautiful, gorgeous, attractive,* and *pretty?*

"I don't need to be gorgeous, but I want to be pretty."

"I feel attractive, but I don't think I'm beautiful."

How are we plastic surgeons, masterful manipulators of mind and matter, to interpret these words thrown so familiarly at us by our patients? Do patients expect us to know what they mean, or judge and decide for them? By stark contrast, straight is straight in any culture and a circle is a circle except at the speed of light.

While attending a meeting of predominantly Caucasian plastic surgeons, one Asian doctor pointed out that Asian, and not Caucasian, definitions of beauty should be the gold standard since there are far more Asian people than there are Caucasians in the world. That ethnocentric view of the norm did not win over the room despite the nervous laughter that followed. It so happened that this doctor was Japanese, so being Chinese, I was wondering what sort of Asian he was talking about. I mused if he thought himself a more handsome Asian as a Japanese man than I might feel as a Chinese. One thing was for sure: I didn't look like him at all.

When a patient seeks "youth" or strives to be "attractive," non-surgical means (i.e., makeup, hairstyle, fashion, accessories, physique, even diction and vocabulary, as with Pygmalion's Eliza Doolittle) can accomplish a lot. We know this intuitively and by examples all around us. Most things sold to women to keep them young and attractive have nothing to do with surgery. Women practice beauty enhancement daily. They are constantly assessing their makeup and critiquing their haircut or choosing clothing styles and accessories. When they don't, it will show. All this has nothing to do with plastic surgery except that at some point all this non-surgical cosmetic behavior becomes inadequate. Patients will seek something more.

A patient with an outdated hairstyle, non-descript outfit, and unflattering makeup will explain how she wants to look more youthful. She knows she is not a ravishing beauty but could look better. She is perhaps fearful of surgery and a bit apologetic about even being in my office. As she expresses reservations about being able to afford plastic surgery, all I might think of is how much of her goals she could achieve by meeting with a hairstylist, a fashion consultant, and a makeup artist rather than me. She will usually agree with me since I am honest in my opinion. But that is not why she is sitting in front of a plastic surgeon. She is search-ing for something that goes beyond beauty achieved with rouge, blush, and lipstick, beyond youthfulness cut with a cute bob, and beyond elegance created by an haute couture evening dress and diamond earrings. There are tens of thousands of hairstylists, makeup art-ists, and fashion experts working their magic on mil-lions of people every day. You can go into a mall, pay a hundred dollars, and come out looking like a million bucks. But cosmetic surgery patients want something life-changing. They are dissatisfied and unfulfilled with temporary, superficial modifications. They toss and turn within their blemished skin, less-than-ideal bodies, and imperfect facial features like the princess being poked by her annoying pea.

The search really lies behind and beneath the meaning and intent of the words spoken so matter-of-factly. Ironically, and mistakenly, patients and surgeons act as if not knowing the obvious meaning and intent of these commonly used words is confessing stupidity or naiveté.

To paraphrase the age-old question about women and their desires, "What do cosmetic patients want?"

A patient comes in saying, "I just want a *nice* nose." Or, "I want to look like myself, just *better*." Or, "I want to look more *attractive*." When a patient asks to have *natural* breast enlargement, she really doesn't mean *natural*. Natural is what she has but *doesn't* want. What she usually means is *not fake* or not obviously *un*natural. So I then have to ask, just when does an unnatural condition (i.e., implanted breasts) begin to look unnaturally unnatural ("rock in a sock" or melon-like)? Do patients see things as more or less natural or unnatural than the surgeon? The natural look in Los Angeles is really an unnatural look in Poughkeepsie. People are always asking me, "Do you think they're real?" as they nod towards some nearby mammary glands. I usually hesitate because I know they are also judging my opinion as to what I think *nice* is. When patients then bring in pictures to illustrate what they mean by natural, I wonder if we've lost track of what real, nice, and natural used to be and think to myself, "When was the last time they visited Poughkeepsie?"

Besides looking natural or real, there is the issue of acting or feeling natural. This goes beyond the three-dimensional physical and visual description into the fourth dimension of movement or texture. Natural-*looking* breasts can have a very unnatural *feel* and even more unnatural *movement* to them. The same is true with facial rejuvenation where a beautiful static picture does little justice to the unnatural movement, or lack of movement, in real time. In fact, Virginia Blum, in her book *Flesh Wounds: The Culture of Cosmetic Surgery*, criticizes this surgical goal of two-dimensional photo-perfection; surgery shouldn't be judged by, or performed simply for, its appearance in a photo album. As mundane as it sounds, it is not inappropriate for one to ask, "Just what do you mean by *natural* or *better* or *nice?*"

Unfortunately, this is not simply a frivolous game of wordplay and not enough surgeons and patients spend adequate time defining these words. As obsessive and ridiculously frustrating as it can seem to nitpick the meaning of words, the artistic assessment and interpretation for the plastic surgeon begins with the use of language. The use and definition of words beget real decisions regarding real anatomy by real doctors on real patients with real consequences. Breasts with natural movement may require implants on top of the chest muscles while breasts with a more natural feel may demand implants under the muscles. Lack of understanding during the pre-surgical planning phase can lead to real problems and real problems lead to real unhappy patients. In contrast, there is no need for interpretation when someone needs an appendectomy or coronary bypass.

Since communication and interpretation is so crucial to what I do, it always astounds me how some surgeons think they can reach this point of speaking a common language with their patients in such a short period of time. While I admit it is not impossible for instantaneous synchronization of thought, as in the romanticization of lovers meeting for the first time— sort of a love at first thought—it is my experience that the meeting of the minds occurs mainly by force of the plastic surgeon's position as the voice of authority. Real understanding requires time.

In *Flesh Wounds*, Blum has even gone on to suggest that sexual transference and the power of a chauvinistic perspective influence most of the female choices in plastic surgery. That may in part be true, but what of the male patient with the male plastic surgeon or the female patient with the female plastic surgeon? What kind of gender-specific transference and "sexual exploitation" is occurring in these situations? While gender may play a supporting role, it is more likely that the position of authority, as occurs with medically necessary treatment, dis-empowers the patient to think on equal terms.

This position of authority is actually quite important. Surgeons can dictate what they will do with a patient by force of suggestion. It also raises the question of whether a surgeon is using language and words for his or her benefit, for the patient's, or for the common good, as is the heart of true communication. "I can make you look terrific!" may be a statement a surgeon is making about his abilities for his own gratification and also an enticement to commit to a surgical procedure. It may also be uttered to give a patient an all-important emotional boost and encouragement. After all, "looking terrific" is what they are there for. Reverse psychology may be used as in a statement such as, "I'm not sure I can do anything to help you" whereby a clever surgeon may be revealing his limitations while subtly encouraging a disappointed patient to implore him to work his miracles to "save" her. The paternalistic figurehead may seem like a last bastion of hope. Or, he may truly be telling the unfortunate truth. At any rate, truthful verbalization, accurate understanding, and honest discussion between plastic surgeon and patient can only take place over an extended period of time. It certainly will take more than a few minutes one-on-one and not through a go-between consultant.

Words and language are also critical during the peri-operative process. Allowing surgical results to *settle* may mean allowing immediate post-surgical effects, like swelling and tension, to abate. Or it may mean, "Let's give things time to see if an undesirable result will improve"—and let's keep our magical fingers crossed behind our backs. Some surgeries will truly "settle" over time, but others are just an honest exercise in wishful thinking. We can almost visualize the collagen fibers, willing them to stretch and relax, allowing the breast implants to sink into the lower pole of the breast, or we sense the sponginess of the post-mid-facelift edema and, with a form of mental prestidigitation, verbally massage the fluid from the swollen and much-too-prominent cheeks as they ever so imperceptibly deflate into a more normal posture. We think that by saying it, we can induce these things to happen.

Waiting for something to *settle* may also allow valuable time to pass in order for patients themselves to acclimate emotionally to their results. Patients are often too eager to see and assess their results. "Let things settle" we might say as if referring to a personal setback that we know, or hope, will heal itself with the passage of time. Perhaps we are referring to the emotional settling of the patient herself as in "settle down, kids!"

We often tell one patient to wait for the scarring process, or its contraction, to kick in, hopefully to achieve a better look than initially produced, as in superficial or laser liposuction where subcutaneous trauma initiates collagen or scar formation that might lead to a tighter effect. Yet we will tell another patient to wait for the scarring process, in this case, remodeling, to mature, allowing a result that is too tight to loosen. Are the words intended to place some "English" spin on the surgical result much like a golfer or bowler uses body English to mind-control a ball into the hole or towards a pin? Are we using the English language as bait as would a politician casting for votes or a public relations spin-doctor polishing a celebrity's image? We are not necessarily talking out of both sides of the mouth; we may truly want to believe what we say because we are purposefully taking known physiological processes (scar contraction and scar maturation) into differential consideration. It is part truth, part manipulation, part pleading, part stalling, all contributing to the art of medicine. More than half the battle is won if the patient feels better about herself. For many of us, what our parents told us is true: Time, in fact, does heal all wounds, and words can truly help us.

We can talk about *sculpting* or *contouring* a body as if we are Augustin Rodin or Michaelangelo when in fact we are removing large portions of fat and skin in a less than elegant manner like bulldozers moving mountains of mud. *Sculpting* sounds more precise, artistic, and inviting than it may actually be—certainly better than "carving," "slicing," "excising," or "whittling" do. Actually, I do believe I am sculpting a body or face. It just may not look like it at the time.

The words *exotic, Asian,* or *elegant* all evoke positive impressions and can be applied equally to Angelina Jolie, Audrey Hepburn, and Catherine Zeta-Jones or, depending on one's interpretation, to the Cat Woman, an overdone browlift, exaggerated canthopexies, or an excessively tight neckline. An attempt at "*exotic*" may result in simply the "*bizarre.*" Hopefully, *exotic* is what the patient wanted since an ill-timed, unintended slip of the tongue may evoke an unwanted reaction from the patient. This faux pas is possibly worse than the surgery itself since often it is other people's reaction to a patient's surgery that is important, not necessarily the surgery itself. In some cases, it is best to hold one's tongue. As in marriage, learning when *not* to speak can be crucial.

* * *

Plastic surgeons start out in the educational process as mere physicians and surgeons, learning about anatomy, physiology, manipulation of bone, cartilage, skin, and fat, use of alloplastic and autogenous materials, and the history of various aesthetic concepts. We learn to measure human form, name minute anatomical structures, photograph body parts, dictate meticulous operative reports, and explain complex techniques in a precise, scientific, and objective manner, even anointing them with highfalutin monikers such as "modified radical mastectomy," "deep-plane rhytidectomy," "high lateral-tension abdominoplasty," and "transverse rectus abdominus myocutaneous island free flap." Plastic surgery itself can then seem to be precise, scientific, well-defined, and predictable.

Patients can believe that a rhinoplasty will produce a post-operative result that will fit within an absolute classic norm that translates into beauty, as if getting a "nose job" automatically means being more attractive, just like there is only one way for a car to get a lube job. They think that a boob job with a certain breast implant will give a pre-ordained given size, look, and instant sexiness as in "don't go for anything less than three hundreds." They expect that something called a "facelift" will automatically make them look ten years younger but not a different person as in "when I'm fifty, I'm going in for my lift." They hope scars will become invisible.

As plastic surgeons mature, we learn that language is a useful and powerful tool, sometimes more useful and powerful than the surgery itself. Language then needs to be mastered, harnessed, and hopefully cherished, not abused. One obvious example of the importance of language is the informed consent form. This legal document can be minutely scrutinized for inclusions and omissions of key words and phrases. It can be a dispassionate and truthful explanation of what can happen. Alternatively, it can be an exhaustive litany of defensive verbiage designed to pummel a weary brain into hypnotic submission, providing the bulletproof defense against any mishap. Sometimes whether a patient is satisfied with surgery is dependent on if certain words had been discussed pre-operatively and placed in the informed consent document. Hearing an unhappy patient utter the words "you never said…" or "you didn't mention…" can bring a chill to any plastic surgeon's spine. The more extensive the informed consent, the more protected one feels.

How an operative report is dictated should, and can, but often doesn't, convey a precise dramatization of what occurred in the operating room and is another example of the power and importance of words. Each word or phrase can be dissected, examined, and critiqued more meticulously than the actual patient or surgery. One should ideally be able to understand everything that transpired in an operation by reading the operative report. In reality, operative reports vary considerably in their completeness or incompleteness, as the case may be. A typical passage from a face-lift report might read as follows: "The pre-operative markings were incised with the scalpel and the skin was undermined in the usual manner." How deep are we talking? Was it sub-SMAS or subcutaneous? Did he go to the anterior border of the parotid gland or all the way to the nasolabial fold? What is the "usual manner" for this particular surgeon? Was there perfect and uniform thickness throughout? I am reminded of the line in the *Ben Hur* movie script, "And they ran," that the director translated into eight minutes of thrilling, memorable chariot races. Words can be meticulously precise or leave much to one's imagination.

Given the cosmopolitan environment in which many plastic surgeons now work, difficulties lurk just beneath an adjective when consulting with patients in a foreign language or culture. Medical verbiage is alien enough, but in broken Mandarin or Spanish or Farsi, it may be unintelligible. Imagine trying to decide what "beautiful" exactly means to a native of Shandong Province or a member of the Saudi royal family. Believe me, I've been there with patients looking adoringly at me and pleading with great admiration and expectation to give them (translated into English) "*nice-looking*" eyes or a "*better-looking*" face all the while with them glancing at my Harvard diplomas in awe and with me trying to explain to a son or daughter acting as interpreter what the fifth dimension is all about. Sometimes it feels as if we might as well be speaking in animal language.

Contrary to most assumptions, I feel at a disadvantage when consulting with ethnically Asian patients since they often believe that I, as a doctor of Chinese origin, have some magical insight into their desires and somehow expect me to be able to fully understand their point of view just because I am Asian. They are often so respectful of a medical doctor that the use of language is discarded in favor of blind trust because as a highly trained Chinese plastic surgeon with two degrees from Harvard, I should automatically know. But I don't. When they start to try to talk to me in Mandarin, all hell breaks loose. Then my broken Chinese probably makes me sound unintelligent. As we start gesturing with our hands, the power of language becomes quite clear in its absence.

Even conversing in the same language can be downright aggravating and confusing, to which husbands and wives in the same household can attest. Perhaps that is why the art of gesture, attitude, facial expression, and omnipotent silence is perfected in perfect marriages. On the other hand, it is not uncommon for husbands and wives to contradict each other when in consultation for one or the other.

"You told me your eyes *bothered* you."

"I don't mean *bothered*. I just *notice* it."

"You mean it doesn't *bother* you?"

"Well, it does, but not *really* bother me."

"Doc, she complains to me all the time."

"So, I do complain, dear. So what?"

"So, it *does bother* you."

"But not so that I would actually *do* anything about it."

"So why are you *here*, honey?"

Equally disconcerting to me is when one spouse will actually be the mouthpiece for the other, unapologetically putting words into the other's mouth.

"Let me explain how she/he feels. I mean, she's/he's *beautiful/handsome.* You can see. I think she/he is *perfect.* But I think, I mean, she/he thinks there can be some *improvement.* She/he doesn't need a lot, just a *little,* just *enough* to make her/him even *more* beautiful/handsome—but not *too much,* of course. We just want you to make her/him look *naturally enhanced.* She/he wants to look like her/himself. Because, of course, she's/he's *perfect.*"

Of course. Perfect!

* * *

At some time, usually much after their formal medical or surgical education is complete, plastic surgeons learn and utilize words of encouragement and key words evoking positive images in order to rightfully gain their patient's confidence. Sometimes the doctors learn it from their staff. Just as a firm handshake is taught to business school students to be a communication tool, positive language can be used to advantage in easing the patient through the plastic surgical process. As indicated before, positive feedback, positive imagery, and positive words validating patient's feelings are all appropriate methods in assisting patients and physicians through the surgical process. The "laying on of words" can be invaluable.

"You look *terrific*" is encouraging to a patient despite looking like she just fell off a second-story balcony. No one wants to be hear, "Wow, what happened?

You're pretty swollen" three days after surgery, even if they are.

"The implants are starting to *settle*" is reassuring to a patient upset at an unnatural appearance to her augmented breasts when she might wonder why she wanted such big breasts to begin with.

"The change *is wonderfully subtle*" may be code for "there is no discernible improvement" or a genuine compliment for a job well-camouflaged (as requested, of course). At the same time, someone else in the examining room might be thinking to themselves, "How *much* did this surgery cost?"

Contrary to popular belief and usage, *nip, tuck, tweak,* and *lift* are not medical terms but popular colloquial words functioning as both noun and verb to describe physical changes that convey an ill-defined emotional benefit as in "I'm just going in for a little tuck" or "Can you just tweak it a bit?" When a patient asks for a little *nip and tuck,* she usually means a subtle change but also implies little cost. She may not understand that an "*undone*" look often requires more, not less, surgery. "I want just a slight lift" or "Can't you just make the nose a little smaller?" may be like asking to raise the foundation of a three-story Tudor house just an inch or two. It is sometimes harder than just adding a whole new story. Some little surgeries can have more telltale signs of being "*done*" than more comprehensive and extensive surgeries designed to harmonize the anatomy. How to translate these words into action is the challenge of plastic surgery since, as far as I know, there is no specific surgery that has been defined as a nip, or a tuck, or a nip-and-tuck procedure (or a *boob job* or *nose job*). At least I've never learned them.

Patients themselves can inadvertently get into the wordplay game. The intangible world of emotions, feelings, and self-critique can easily conflict with tangible, hard, physical changes demanded by plastic surgery. Patients become a little bit schizophrenic. For example, it is not uncommon for patients to be unhappy about a particular body part and request a change but then add, "I don't want my husband/boyfriend to know" or "I don't want anyone to think I really had plastic surgery done." It is, of course, understandable for a patient to want to gain the benefits of surgery without being a walking advertisement, but meanwhile the plastic surgeon is thinking, *you want a change but you don't want anyone to notice the change. You want to be done but not look done. You want me to touch you and manipulate your tissues without signs of my being there. You certainly don't want to look exactly the same after paying all that money... unless you want something really subtle.* Now that's tricky to interpret.

Psycho-emotional feelings about oneself as manifested by a physical structure have to be translated into words that then are accurately interpreted by the plastic surgeon. The difference between being "The Best!" and being a "butcher" to a patient is often an invisibly thin line of verbiage. Maybe we should just tell prospective patients they look "*fabulous*" and "*extraordinary*," hope they agree, and forego the surgery altogether. Life might be simpler!

Because cosmetic surgery is a highly competitive field, advertising, taboo for years, is now commonplace, even rampant, with ad after ad falling over themselves in every imaginable media outlet. Advertising has been necessary because cosmetic surgery is unnecessary. Necessary things don't need to be advertised.

When is the last time you saw an advertisement for air or postage stamps or electricity? Most advertisements are a combination of visual images and the use of carefully chosen language. As opposed to informational advertising that simply provides data or information, such as education, hospital affiliation, or procedures performed, persuasive or marketing advertisement seeks to motivate patients into action or change their behavior, to somehow sway them to use the advertiser.

"Artistic" is a popular adjective used by many cosmetic surgeons in their advertisements to describe themselves or their surgery. It implies creativity, lofty values, and extraordinary knowledge of the elements of beauty: something deeper than just cutting and sewing. But what does it really mean and say about the surgeon? Is he a sculptor or a painter? Does playing the piano count more or less in being artistic than drawing portraits or writing sonnets? Can one be artistic without having any artistic talents? Does it matter? Does he have an extraordinary eye for beauty? While all plastic and cosmetic surgeons believe they possess such innate judgment for feminine beauty, nine out of ten guys sitting at a bar with peanuts and a two-dollar bottle of beer will attest to having the same sort of eye. Does he know classic Greco-Roman concepts of beauty, the Golden Proportion, and essential facial and body anatomy? One would expect so. Is he apt to look at human form in a Picasso-esque, Ruben-esque, or Dali-esque manner?

I use *artistic* both as a tangible and intangible adjective. When I was a young musician playing the violin, it was soon evident that good music had elements of technicality and musicality. They were interdependent yet also mutually exclusive. A violinist can be technically brilliant but display no musicality or emotion. You just knew when someone wasn't artistic. You could, unfortunately, hear it. Conversely, one can have great feeling for the music but not be technically precise. That was my curse as a budding violinist. I was a bit more right-brain dominant than left-brain proficient. Many singers have that quality. They sing out of tune but convey deep feeling and sensitivity—so, too, self-taught musicians. Bob Dylan, Rod Stewart, and jazz musicians come to mind. Really great music usually has both. Like beauty, you can sense artistic qualities but may not be able to define them.

Being artistic, or possessing the ability to create art, is also, and perhaps more importantly, a process, and not a specific technique. It is this more tangible meaning that may lend greater significance to the description "artistic": the *artistic process.* How a plastic surgeon views and interprets his subject is as important as how well he separates tissue planes. How sensitive he is to the inner mind and soul of his patients is as crucial as what implants, fillers, and sutures he uses. How he projects the emotional changes the patient is subconsciously expecting is equally critical as how fast he can perform surgery or how deft he is with an endoscope. Establishing the artistic *process* and being true to it may make the *making* of the art easier. How a surgeon analyzes anatomy, establishes specific goals, and plans and executes precise technical maneuvers is just part of the *artistic* process. You can teach the *artistic process,* but not teach how to be artistic.

The tools of communication and interpretation, and of manipulating and shaping the result, are in the language and the words. How well and accurately a cosmetic surgeon masters these tools when treating a patient is critical to how he uses his surgical tools. Imagine what would happen if a patient and surgeon never talked! The end point is not the doing of the surgery itself, though that is how plastic surgeons earn their living. Neither is it the anatomic transformation that is achieved, though that is what a patient may desire. They are not the goals any more than the end result is the word on the page in literature or the notes on the staff in music or the oil on the canvas in paintings. Each of those is merely the vehicle or the medium by which one's existence is somehow hopefully enhanced. Rather, it is the psycho-emotional state within a person created by the surgery, the word, the note, and the paint that is the true goal. For most purchases we make, we can point to what we want in a store, pay for it, take it home, and enjoy it without uttering a sound. But what we look for in art, music, literature, and plastic surgery is to be *moved*, to be *inspired*, to be *provoked*, and to make life more *meaningful* and *enjoyable*. It is to get beyond the tangibles that the words we utter seem to imply and to feel and live the meaning and intent of the words and phrases. It is to find the truth in the phrase, "Life is beautiful." It is for one to feel *beautiful* or *attractive* or *gorgeous* or *youthful* or *exotic* or *fabulous* or *fantastic*.

While words are necessary, they may not be sufficient and the words we choose may hurt or help the application and the outcome of the artistic process.

CHAPTER 11:

HYPE, HYPE...HOORAY???

Question: What's the difference between
a plastic surgeon and God?

Answer: God doesn't believe He is a plastic surgeon.

"Abstract art, a product of the untalented sold by the unprincipled to the utterly bewildered."
—*Al Capp, cartoonist*

* * *

Plastic surgery is an art form, but it is also a medical industry comprised of surgical professionals known to be especially innovative and entrepreneurial. Inventions and marketing go hand-in-hand in most other fields of business but are often suspect when blatantly promoted in the actual practice of medicine. Advances in medicine are usually intended for the benefit of the common good as well as the individual patient. As a specialty that transcends the confines of the ivory tower of academia and that unabashedly utilizes the media to unveil the mysteries of its inner workings to the general public, widely disseminated information in the loudest form can be its lifeblood.

"The times, they are a-changin"; one often might think, *He who toots the loudest, wins.*

Since its birth, and certainly since my nascent interest in plastic surgery as a third-year medical student at Harvard Medical School in 1977, plastic surgery has been a field devoted to problem solving. Whether it is developing a way of repairing the euphemistic "harelip" over two thousand years ago in China, or recreating a semblance of a nose from tissues of the forehead in India a millennium ago, or imagining a method of transferring skin of the arm to replace missing skin of the nose in Italy during the sixteenth century, anatomical problems beget solutions that someone, not always the innovator, will popularize and perpetuate. It is not so much the learning of how to perform a well-delineated and step-wise surgical procedure that distinguishes plastic surgeons, but, rather, how cleverly or rationally one can solve an individual anatomical or functional problem. I didn't find learning "how to do a gallbladder" or memorizing the boundaries of a modified radical mastectomy very stimulating. While seemingly the goal of general surgical education, I didn't want to repeat the same operation over and over again the same way on every single patient. I wanted to learn how to solve anatomical and functional puzzles. I thought that dreaming up customized solutions for individual patients was infinitely more interesting, challenging, and rewarding for me and whatever artistic qualities I possessed at the time. Plastic surgery as an intellectual, spatial, anatomical, and creative endeavor fit me like skin on a well-toned body.

In my first year as the token Chinese resident in plastic surgery at the University of Miami, I remember performing a double rotation flap closure of a spinal wound, resulting in a yin-yang design. I thought it was simultaneously rather clever, practical, and attractive, and it began my quest for plastic surgery as an artistic endeavor rather than merely a technical challenge. Another patient who lost one half of the lower face to cancer treatment required a large flap from the chest as well as an even larger flap from the back in a marathon twenty-two-hour procedure. At that time, it was a first-of-its-kind combination and an unenviable record for the Miami Veterans' Administration hospital.

In private practice, there was a middle-aged woman with a cancer of the bridge of the nose who serendipitously also had a large, droopy, and rather unattractive nose that I was able to make more attractive at the same time as curing the cancer, thus erasing the stigma of having cancer at all. I also began to use a method of increasing the projection of the nose utilizing the existing cartilages of the nose without the usual grafts or implants, an approach I "discovered" having seen problems with the latter methods. As a member of a newly formed breast center, I tried, rather unsuccessfully, to entice cancer surgeons, radiation therapists, and oncologists to think outside their usual box and to convince them that the treatment of breast cancer should incorporate concepts of breast enhancement. I believe that cancer patients can potentially look better coming out of treatment than when they go in, on par with non-cancer patients having purely cosmetic breast surgery. I was even bold (or ignorant) enough to suggest that plastic surgeons should be the captain of the cancer team, only to watch a cross-town center advertise "oncoplastic" treatment of breast cancer as a selling point a decade later. Much of these individual innovations were a direct application of principles, not techniques, expounded by my mentor, Dr. Millard, in his book *Principlization of Plastic Surgery*: Imagination Sparks Innovation, Principle #26; Avoid the Rut of Routine, Principle #25; Think while Down and Turn Setback into Victory, Principle #27, etc.

Of course, one plastic surgeon cannot possibly solve all of the problems and concerns of all the potential patients. My experience is not unique and is almost expected of well-trained plastic surgeons. As a group, plastic surgeons and their related technological and professional supports develop and produce numerous devices, inventions, techniques, maneuvers, modifications, and gadgets that get disseminated to other plastic surgeons and the general public through innumerable professional and lay-media outlets. What to do with all these innovations?

The variety of things I have "discovered" that help me treat patients are not things I have learned in my training or in continuing medical education courses or even through discourse with my fellow plastic surgeons. They are things that I have thought out rationally or have stumbled upon. Much of the process for me is simply rational thinking based on principles taking into consideration logic and anatomy. At times I am too busy (or perhaps too lazy?) to research all the techniques published that address issues in question. I have no illusions that these things are revolutionary, optimal, or even original, but they do work for me and I have "discovered" them within the confines of my own operating room and creative thought process. Many have germinated from reconstructive efforts that then get applied to cosmetic patients. This is, in fact, much the history of the "unnecessary" cosmetic surgery being built on the foundation of necessary reconstructive surgery.

Craniofacial surgeons were dissecting faces in an extended deep plane to reassemble pediatric and adult facial structures long before cosmetic applications gave life to endoscopic, deep-plane, and subperiosteal lifts so prevalent today. Aggressively moving large areas of tissues to heal wounds throughout the body has helped establish the science and field of total body contouring based on the superficial fascial system and perforator anatomy. The most popular cosmetic medical treatment in America today is the use of Botox, the world's most potent neurotoxin, originally used to treat blepharospasm and strabismus.

Like me, some plastic surgeons pass their ideas on to other doctors informally to be adopted or discarded as they see fit. Most are just part of one's private "bag of tricks" because most plastic surgeons practice by choice in a private setting without the glare of the media. A choice few of these thousands of innovations truly revolutionize the thinking or practice of plastic surgery. These advances include tissue expanders (inflatable balloons placed under tissue to stretch and create new skin, as occurs with extreme weight gain and pregnancy), silicone breast implants that are the gold standard for prosthetic breast augmentation (in spite of all their controversies), liposuction that evolved from a relatively crude concept of scraping fat with a curette, and endoscopic procedures that borrowed from other surgical specialties (such as gastrointestinal surgery, orthopedic surgery, and otolaryngology) the idea of operating through scopes to magnify vision and limit incision length.

The push to make an impact on our profession and on our patients is driven partly by humanism and partly by ego, and more often now by financial gain. We feel the need to help our patients...as well as ourselves. The stage we perform on is usually small and confined to our hospital, office, or immediate practice community. But there are many plastic surgeons who thrive under the glow of a television camera or revel in the black-and-white relief of monthly newsstand magazines or who subscribe to the "whole world is a stage" philosophy. Certainly businesses that cater to the plastic surgery industry, like those involved in topical skin care, anti-aging formulations, laser, ultrasonic, radio frequency, or intense pulsed light machine manufacturing, implantable and injectable materials, and specialized surgical tools and instruments, all require media exposure on a concentrated and constant level to survive and thrive. Because of the fertile ground for innovation and the link between exposure and success, hype is a good thing for the business of plastic surgery and publicity can be the key to success for a plastic surgeon. As one notoriously well-known plastic surgeon joked, "There's no such thing as bad publicity!" in a quote borrowed from early twentieth-century Irish dramatist Brendan Behan. If so, the idea is to keep the hype going on a constant level. If patients don't know your name, they can't call you.

The conflicts between medicine as a humanistic endeavor and medicine as a for-profit business become more intense each day and the yin and yang of life is never more evident as in the push and pull of innovation and marketing in plastic surgery. Some surgeons carry self-promotion to an extreme by attempting to patent procedures or by repackaging established procedures or techniques, and subsequently claim to be original innovators or inventors of something new and revolutionary. There are many ways of spinning loose old facts into spools of modern gold. Of course, no one should begrudge a doctor, even a plastic surgeon, the right to earn a comfortable living. It is more the methodology and motivation that is in question given the explosion of the media industry. Word of individual mouth is being eclipsed by word of mass print or online broadcast. Public relation ploys and advertising are favored over brick-by-brick practice building.

In the early days of my career in the late-1980s, the local university plastic surgery division drafted me to present the "con" side of a debate between those who believed advertising in medicine, and specifically plastic surgery, was appropriate, and those who didn't. Advertising, originally taboo for medical doctors, had begun its trend toward being widely practiced, uniformly acceptable, and frequently necessary. Informational ads in the yellow pages had been largely replaced by self-promoting ads in mass media outlets designed to entice, convince, and motivate prospective patients into action. The simple listing of practice location, phone number, educational training, and scope of expertise does not create nearly the impact on the general public as glossy pictorials with stunningly beautiful models, glowing testimonials, and price discounts.

I argued that a plastic surgeon's career is broadly divided into three traditional phases. In the beginning of his career, coming out from residency training, a surgeon needs to establish a track record in his hospitals and communities by "putting in his dues" before he can make legitimate claims that set himself apart from other surgeons. That means hitting the emergency rooms for trauma cases in the middle of the night that often require long hours of reconstructive surgery at near or actual pro bono rates of remuneration. It is the tradition of all surgical specialties so everyone begins their practice on a level playing field.

In the middle part of his career, when he should be at the height of his productivity, a surgeon should have established a certain standing and referral network in the community by the success of his past work, thus obviating a need for advertising. Trust and business is "earned," not bought. Doing good work on patients of other doctors ensures future referrals from those grateful and impressed doctors. Good doctors tend to "hang," professionally that is, with other good doctors. This was definitely the modus operandus my father used during his neurosurgical career in the 1960s, '70s, and '80s, and was the strategy I defaulted to as I began my career in the late 1980s and '90s. If I took excellent care of a doctor's patients and achieved laudable results, I benefited from his or her entire practice. His patients, in turn, hopefully benefited from my dedication and expertise.

Finally, I argued, in the "twilight" of his career, the successful surgeon who felt the "need" to advertise might be thought of as self-promoting, driven by ego (seeing his name in print or on television and, thus, being famous) or greed (as if a good income and comfortable living standard weren't satisfying enough), while those who were less successful were advertising because perhaps their work wasn't satisfactory to their own patients. Ergo, no one really needed to advertise if they did good work. Often this is true in real life:

The more successful and respected you are, the less the public sees you in paid advertisements.

In the constant push for innovation, the demand of finding practical solutions to everyday problems is balanced by the fear of failure. This is the inevitable internal debate between the pros and cons, the advantages and the disadvantages, the benefits and the risks of surgical, or non-surgical, intervention. One wants the cure without doing harm. One wants to be in the forefront of one's profession for fear of being out of sight, outdated, or obsolete. One wants to be thought of the most advanced, up-to-date expert and not the old-fashioned, behind-the-times old fogey. One wants to be known for being in the know rather than in the dark or out of the loop. One wants the money in the bag rather than a day late and a dollar short.

Yet the risk of being the "first on the block" is that you are the first to demonstrate the ineffectiveness, or even the dangers, of something new. In the competitiveness of being the discoverer of America, one can end up discovering a barren, soon-to-be-forgotten island on which one dies without ever seeing America. Instead of providing the cure for cancer, one can be accused of hawking snake oil, as in the case of the drug Laetrile, made famous by actor Steve McQueen in his battle against mesothelioma. The use of foam sponges for breast augmentation, ivory, paraffin, and various metals for nasal reconstruction, and liquid silicone for cosmetic facial and breast enhancement all had their proponents in their heyday and all have since been abandoned or vilified by the mainstream medical establishment. Certainly there is a culture of "nothing ventured, nothing gained" in plastic surgery, but the prevalence and power of the media and the possibility of worldwide, not only around-the-block, fame and fortune has magnified the do-or-die stakes.

In Beverly Hills, the indisputable mecca of plastic surgery, who doesn't want to be known as the plastic surgeon to the stars? The drive is so strong that eventually everyone does, or can, claim that moniker. One can have some of the most famous, or infamous, faces show up in his office without really trying. Who doesn't want to be known as the innovator of the latest hot procedure? Instead of disseminating knowledge like doctors and educators do, one can be accused of self-aggrandizement or greediness. Fame and fortune should be byproducts of professional goals, not the goals themselves.

Medicine as a whole is becoming, or has become, the possession of the general public. Demand and knowledge have driven medicine to produce products, devices, and procedures that the public desires, from time-release capsules requiring less frequent dosing, to less destructive ablative or extirpative procedures, to lighter-weight, waterproof casting materials, to medication that will make hair grow, maintain erections, smooth skin wrinkles, and lighten skin tone. Direct advertising by drug manufacturers often compels doctors to fill prescriptions at a patient's request as the public becomes armed with the knowledge previously reserved for the doctors themselves. Yet there are also questionable products that claim, without scientific verification, to make cellulite disappear, promote sexual drive, increase bust size, and, yes, make hair grow, maintain erections, smooth skin wrinkles, and lighten skin tone!

Information about any of these products, most probably, is not found in various peer-reviewed professional journals that a few thousand doctors read but, rather, in glossy, ad-saturated, self-promoting, aromatic lifestyle periodicals that many more millions of readers and potential patients buy. Often these lay-publications or mass media outlets will carry a plastic surgery-related "fact," or quasi-fact, before the professional journals disseminate it. Peer-reviewed articles can take months or even years to be widely known, whereas the general public may learn of a new product or procedure even before the plastic surgeon.

I have often been quizzed by patients about something they heard about before the medical community has had a chance to evaluate it. Plastic surgeons have been influenced to see what their patient population is reading even if it is too "glossy" or "girly" to be seen with it out in full public view. Thus I am forced to peruse *Glamour, Cosmopolitan, Elle,* and even *OK!* and *US Weekly* in the protected privacy of the inner sanctum of my medical office. More often than not, the hype out in the real world is introduced to a befuddled plastic surgeon before he or she even realizes there is hype. This occurred with "teenage surgery," "husband-wife surgery," "belly-button beautification," and "lunch-time facelifts."

I remember a reporter calling to question me about what I thought about the teenage rhinoplasty fad that was sweeping the nation. I asked my two colleagues with whom I shared an office at the time if they were aware of this fad. They weren't. More recently, a laser company touted the benefits of their skin-tightening machine by quoting the *New York Post* that called it the "Best Quality-of-life Breakthrough" for wrinkles. Imagine promoting a medical device because of an endorsement from *the New York Post*!!!

A plastic surgeon can stimulate hype, promote hype, participate in hype, shun hype, or criticize and refute hype. His actions will reveal his inner nature, can help him succeed, or can destroy his practice. The same can be said for the plastic surgery profession as a whole. Hype and its promise of fame and fortune can be hard to resist, like the siren call of sex, drugs, and rock and roll. Not uncommonly, a doctor caught up in all this hype can end up front-page news as a prelude to a lengthy jail sentence, or worse.

Our national plastic surgery organization is so aware of this hyped-up, publicity-crazed, media-driven environment that it has educational courses on what a plastic surgeon should do when local media calls. While some plastic surgeons may be content with working quietly in the confines of private operating rooms, the fact is the media needs stories! They are as much experts at selling sound bites and magnifying minutiae as they are in educating the public and disseminating truth and useful knowledge.

The fact is that plastic surgery, once the kingdom of socialites and movie stars, has truly come to the masses and the masses are coming to it. Competition, credit cards, and credit companies catering to cosmetic surgery patients have made plastic surgery available to almost everyone, albeit at different levels of expertise and safety. So-called common folks, whomever that might indicate, contemplate their appearance and contour no matter where they live. Facial wrinkles are just as irritating to a housewife in Iowa as to a matron in Miami. Fat on the thighs is as undesirable in Pacoima as it is in Paris. Full breasts are as sexy to young women, and men, in a honky-tonk town as they are in Hollywood. Avon sells beauty on the Great Wall of China as well as on Wall Street. *Elle, Glamour,* and *Cosmopolitan* are just as easily found in a grimy newsstand in urban Detroit as in the boutique shops at upscale W or Four Seasons hotels in Tokyo and London. Ads for plastic surgery are found on AOL Internet sites, talk radio, and the local town-crier newspaper. The desire, the allure, and the gossip of plastic surgery are ubiquitous.

One of the more recently "hyped" technological advances was ultrasonic liposuction. The idea was that ultrasonic waves emitted by a wand-like suction cannula inserted under the skin could selectively emulsify fat cells similar to the ultrasonic lithotripsy of kidney stones. The emulsion could then be removed by suction. The procedure was touted to be quicker, safer, gentle, and more selective than regular vacuum liposuction. The idea was quite attractive on paper and experts in the new field were highlighting the benefits in women's magazine and the lay-press much before critical studies or adequate experience was obtained. Many advantages were true and various companies that manufactured the machines figured prominently in keeping the topic in front of the public. Soon prospective patients were proactively seeking out surgeons who performed this technique. Of course, only the surgeons who were testing the technique had the equipment to perform the procedure. Some took advantage of this by marketing the procedure directly to the public. The public loves anything new and technologically advanced, reflexively equating it with "better."

Initially, everyday plastic surgeons were unarmed with the tools and the knowledge. Patients could only get the procedure from those with access to the technology. Unbeknownst to them, many experts doubted the superiority of the method over traditional liposuction techniques or used the machine sparingly for only a few seconds to "soften" or "loosen" the fat. They mainly relied on machine vacuum to do most of the fat extraction. Patients were still thinking they were getting unique, high-tech, ultrasonic liposuction.

As more plastic surgeons felt the heat of competition, more began to purchase the ultrasonic equipment and more procedures were performed. While experience and technology began to improve, it became clear that the procedure was not all that improved over traditional vacuum liposuction and some of the initial claims of improved results or less bruising and swelling were not that impressive. Because there was a learning curve to the technique that every plastic surgeon had to experience firsthand, there were increased risks of collateral damage. The incidence of over-treatment, as well as the significant costs of the procedure, quickly made ultrasonic liposuction the hype of the past. It left a number of unfortunate patients injured in its path. Seroma rates were higher and injury to the skin occurred more frequently than with traditional non-ultrasonic liposuction.

A recent survey among plastic surgeons revealed that about 25 percent use ultrasonic liposuction in some form or fashion in their practice, indicating that some still find the application useful, but certainly not revolutionary. The natural history of plastic surgical innovation often follows the well-known Gartner's Hype Cycle originated by Jackie Fenn, an analyst who described the course of technological advances. Initial inflated expectations, when hype is at its peak, are followed by disillusionment, then enlightenment, and, finally, a plateau of productivity where the advances find their ultimate utility. The problem with the path from expectations to productivity in hyped plastic surgery is that people and lives can be harmed. People often sense the urgency and desire to ride the initial upsurge and promise. Who doesn't want to be the beneficiary of the "latest and greatest"?

Cosmetic surgery is uniquely and precariously positioned in proximity to a murky washbasin of overstatement into which prospective patients can fall between the time- and test-honored predictability of scientific examination and fact, and the temporally myopic, market-driven hyperbole of inflated promise and barely legal claims of miracle cures, all because there is no third-party interposed between patient and doctor. Fat-busting creams, breast-enlarging gadgets, face-lifting exercises have all seen their days. There is no absolute arbiter of truth. Even the FDA (Federal Drug Administration) may have no jurisdiction over many of these products and even when they do, as in the case of collagen and Botox, off-label use is driven by public demand.

Because cosmetic surgery is unnecessary, there should be a tempered response to hype. Treatments or procedures are not required to save lives. Risks of the unknown must be measured against the risks of discontent and the benefits of increased health to otherwise healthy patients. As opposed to medical advances in treating diseases where lack of treatment may run the risk of death, loss of function, or advancement of disease, lack of treatment has no risk, other than psycho-emotional (that, of course, cannot be entirely discounted) in the basically healthy and "well" cosmetic surgery individual.

My own practical approach to new technology and procedures is to examine the scientific basis for the claim and not the potential for patient desire or practice profit. The fact that patients want or like something and that one can make a profit is not a sufficient reason for doctors to provide it. Otherwise, we should be drug-dealers or fast-food franchisees. We need to be held to a higher standard. I also resist the lure of being the first on the block and like to see clinical validation of results: Rather right than first, I say. It is the surgeon in me who wants to see visible and verifiable effects of treatment. If something can be validated, there will be plenty of time and opportunity to utilize it in elective situations. Stem cell therapies for cosmetic purpose will undoubtedly fall into this category.

Of course, my approach is not necessarily the right, or even the most popular, approach. It is just a reflection of my training, education, personality, and philosophy. Plenty of doctors will gush enthusiasm for things at the first mention of the word "new" and "revolutionary," and they may, in fact, be right. Most prudent, science-based practitioners, however, are slow to embrace change without significant skepticism. In some ways, cosmetic surgical behavior mimics a doctor's reputation in investments. The conventional wisdom that doctors are the worst investors parallels their stereotype as professionals with the worst penmanship. The practice of medicine is a slow, arduous task requiring discipline, patience, and a certain degree of marching to a common beat on a well-defined path. Investing in risky ventures, scribbling indecipherably, and following the aroma of hype may be a way to counter such inherent conservatism.

My experience with the hit ABC television show *Extreme Makeover*, the ground-breaking show that subsequently spawned a host of other plastic surgery shows and an entire industry of reality shows, revealed a direct conflict between my medical instincts and the hype of primetime TV. At first skeptical of my own participation, I was encouraged by the executive producer that I would be a good representative of the profession. The more reluctant I was, the more he encouraged me to participate. I relented when there was the promise that future shows would highlight true extreme makeovers of reconstructive patients. Subsequently, and to the producer's credit, one of the first subjects with a reconstructive issue profiled on the show was a patient with a cleft lip and palate on whom I performed a cleft lip rhinoplasty and lip revision. A number of reconstructive cases followed. However, presenting an entertaining show that compressed six or eight hours of concentrated surgery into one or two minutes and six weeks of post-operation recovery into five or ten minutes of airtime interspersed with makeup, hairstyling, exercise routines, and clothes shopping made it all seem too easy and routine. The dramatic makeovers showcased in the weekly "reveals" often exaggerated the surgical results since all the cumulative effects of fashion, cosmetology, and photography were geared toward the most dramatic before-and-after changes.

Although the surgical results alone might have still been camera-worthy, it was obvious that the producers and surgeons specifically selected these patients for their potential for eye-popping transformations and heartfelt stories. This successful formula immediately produced a wave of publicity for individual plastic surgeons and the profession in general. Expectations from patients and of plastic surgeons to produce life- and body-changing makeovers often pushed the bounds of reality and safety. A lot of good came from this exposure for our profession and for patients emboldened by some of the stories and results. Yet it is with a responsible filtering of all the intrinsic hype that this experience must be viewed in real life and in real time. Time-lapsed, couch-safe cosmetic surgery does not exist.

The advantage that plastic surgeons and cosmetic patients have regarding all the hype is that very few of the concerns (i.e., small breasts, facial sagging, fat bulges, and the like) and the technologies are critical for one's health. By definition, the elective nature of cosmetic surgery allows time and experience to be one's ally; neither patient, nor the surgeon, needs to experiment with procedures much before their time. Uncertainty, risks, and purported benefits of a hyped procedure can be effectively weighed against the seriousness of a patient's concern. Patients may feel the persistent pressures of Father Time or the unrelenting effects of Mother Nature but we are usually not talking about life and death matters, or even matters of functionality. Optimal cosmetic surgery candidates are ideally healthy, confident, stable, and productive individuals.

One everyday example is in the treatment of surgical scars. Scars go through a series of physiological events that manifest themselves as changes in quality and characteristics of those scars. Scars can become thick, or raised, or red, or discolored as the so-called inflammatory and proliferative phase of healing takes place. Most scars will end up quite acceptable as they mature and "settle." Unfortunately, the availability of laser treatment of scars, the public desire to speed the process of healing, and the public attraction to such technologically advanced modalities often lead to premature, overly aggressive, and potentially harmful use since it can stimulate just the scarring it was designed to treat; if only one could be more patient...

The cry of "caveat emptor," or "buyer beware," is never more applicable than in the use of hyped products, technologies, or procedures. Cosmetic surgery, like any good science, has its method of utilizing prospective, double-blind studies to test the effect or lack of effect of claims. It is only because there is an ever hungry and vigilant media and an equally ever vigilant public that hype is even a factor in this particular consumer-influenced branch of medicine.

A recent article in the *Clinics of Dermatology* journal underscores the fact that scientific studies on dermatological consumer products, like moisturizers and soaps, are often manipulated by manufacturers and advertisers to hype a certain desirable characteristic or benefit that enhanced the marketability of a product.[9] One example of this is seen in the sale of everyday consumer food items and the concern for salt, whereby a particular brand of bacon is marketed as "low salt," completely ignoring the fat content it possesses. A cereal product labeled as "*no-added* salt" discounts the regular normally high salt content. Food that ordinarily contains a miniscule amount of salt is hyped as no-salt. I once saw a bag of rice advertised prominently as no-salt rice

---

9 Wolf,R, Orion E., Davidovic, B., Skin care products and subtle data manipulation, *Clinics in Dermatology* 2007;25(2)222-224

(normally about five milligrams per half cup). That makes as much sense as no-rice salt.

Undoubtedly there will be a wealth of good that can emerge from all this stimulation and innovation, as our profession and the public can attest. The level of plastic surgery competence and the advances made in improving cosmetic surgical results is, in many ways, a byproduct of the sifting through of the wheat of hyped goods and services and the discarding of the chaff of disappointment and failures. But no one wants to be part of the chaff.

A final note on hype: Hype is not only employed for products, technologies, and services, but for surgeons themselves. Listing, or even marketing, education credentials and achievements is one thing. Advertising in medicine, long taboo, is now widely practiced, accepted, and even considered necessary. But exaggerating claims of being sole originators, inventors, or innovators of procedures is usually, although not always, hype. More often, certain surgeons are popularizers or marketers of techniques. Usually there is not one surgeon definitively revolutionizing a procedure but a collection of collaborative efforts on the part of many. A "revolutionary advance" may be more a gradual evolution or reapplication of an existing technique. With the media so heavily involved in promoting and reporting on plastic surgery, it is also not uncommon for plastic surgeons to highlight their participation in television programs or claim to be stars of this or that show—all well and good. Paid public relations agents may be behind this strategy because one can ride hype all the way to the bank. Hooray!

Plastic surgeons on television shows typically just happen to be in the right place at the right time and serve the producer's needs. Often we are interchange-able as far as the producers go and exposure is more a product of good public relation representation than newsworthy achievement. Promotion is not the same as information. Promotion is designed to motivate action. Claims of imagined stardom are not the same as stardom itself. It is not like having a concerto com-missioned for you because you are Yo Yo Ma or having an entire movie marketed and designed to your exact specifications because you are Steven Spielberg.

Most reputable plastic surgeons will play down their role in the media because use of *too* much hype in promoting oneself is often closely linked to overblown ego or a need to market. One magazine advertisement refers to a local plastic surgeon as "internationally renowned." Based on what? Being *known* and having *renown* are two very different char-acteristics. Another ad calls a different surgeon a "pioneer," despite the fact that the advertiser is not even trained in plastic surgery. Not always, but for the most part, respect within the ranks of the plastic sur-gery profession is inversely related to the volume and hyperbole of the advertisement.

Unfortunately the public responds to spotlights like flies to a light bulb and, like television shows them-selves, the light bulbs just get bigger and brighter. Pretty soon, the airwaves are jumbled with trends that do not exist, products that don't deliver, and surgeons who believe they are more important than their patients. I joke that plastic surgery shows could be about nar-cissistic patients but are now just as likely to be about narcissistic doctors. All this ego-boosting attention can certainly disorient the most well-intended doctor. I remember walking across a parking lot in Beverly

Hills during the height of the *Extreme Makeover* craze when out of the dark night a voice yelled, "Hey, that's Dr. Yuan of *Extreme Makeover!*" I waved at the group of girls who thought they actually saw a celebrity and chuckled with my kids and their friends as we giggled our way toward the ice cream counter at our local drug store. I was amazed that they even cared about seeing this doctor (I wasn't an actor, athlete, or musician), and even more surprised that they recognized me since all Chinese look alike, don't we?

The lengths a plastic surgeon will go to in maintaining a presence in the spotlight is at times humorous. Just like journalists interviewing other journalists about what another journalist said about a newsworthy person, there are often comments by doctors about the work of other doctors. Sometimes there are comments about work that might or might not have been performed on a celebrity the commentator has never seen or treated.

I was entertained by the headlines of a gossip magazine that announced so-and-so's "Fabulous Plastic Surgery!" referring directly to my patient who happened to be one of the world's most recognizable entertainer and who had undergone a complete facial rejuvenation. At first I was afraid that some opportunistic individual had leaked this confidential information. Or perhaps it was the patient who was unapologetic about surgery. I quickly leafed through the magazine and found the article that, instead of reporting on facts, had interviewed another plastic surgeon, whom I personally knew, about what this celebrity *might* have had done. Not only did this doctor speculate on the surgery that *might* have occurred, he even gave laudatory marks to the quality of the work, *if* it had been done. Of course, neither the interviewer nor the plastic surgery commentator knew what truly had transpired. I was pleased that they could give such high marks to the work without knowing if the work had actually been performed. One thing it did besides speculate was to get the other plastic surgeon's name in print: a clever and crafty bit of public relations hype.

Whenever I receive a magazine's request to comment on someone's plastic surgery, I respectfully decline. It is silly and potentially misleading, like speculation masquerading as science. When a patient brings to my attention a spectacular news item or a revolutionary new procedure advertised by a surgeon, I often warn them, "Beware the media. It's the business of the art as much as it is the art of the business." Hype is still hype and time, indeed, will tell.

CHAPTER 12:

COSMETIC VS. RECONSTRUCTIVE

"I'm glad you do reconstruction. I'd never go to someone who only does cosmetic surgery."
—A patient

"I don't think someone who does mostly reconstructive surgery would be as good as someone who does only cosmetic surgery."
—Another patient

* * *

The public's perception of reconstructive and cosmetic surgery is that they are mutually exclusive subspecialties, that somehow they are distinctly different, and that the surgeons practicing each are diametrically opposed. The first patient's statement alludes to a perception that a cosmetic surgeon is not as well-trained as a reconstructive surgeon or is perhaps too superficial in his thinking. The second patient's comment suggests that a reconstructive surgeon can't be a very good cosmetic surgeon because he or she is not specialized, meticulous, or beauty-conscious enough. There is also confusion about the difference between "plastic surgeons" and "cosmetic surgeons" and their usual training.

In a study commissioned by the Plastic Surgery Education Campaign, nearly 90 percent of survey participants who were seriously considering plastic surgery did not understand that anyone with a medical license could perform plastic surgery. While these respondents believed plastic surgeons were the most qualified to perform cosmetic surgery, they were just as likely to choose someone who called himself a cosmetic surgeon, whether or not he was a plastic surgeon. It is confusing even for plastic surgeons since cosmetic surgeons may or may not be trained as plastic surgeons, although most plastic surgeons prefer to be known as plastic surgeons rather than cosmetic surgeons. Some cosmetic surgeons may be gynecologists, general surgeons, or even urologists. Many are non-surgically trained dermatologists or even dentists. Additionally, plastic surgeons may choose to call or not call themselves cosmetic surgeons so there is nothing inherently wrong with being called a cosmetic surgeon or not being called a cosmetic surgeon. You really have to look carefully behind the label and read the fine print as to education and experience. The key thing for a plastic surgeon is whether or not he is certified by the American Board of Plastic Surgery, not necessarily what he calls himself.

Battle lines are drawn between fully trained, board-certified plastic surgeons who do cosmetic surgery and doctors who *call* themselves cosmetic surgeon but may not be plastic surgeons, as well as between fully trained, board-certified plastic surgeons who *only* do cosmetic surgery and fully trained, board-certified plastic surgeons who do cosmetic surgery *and* reconstructive surgery. Now, even I am confused.

A slightly different issue is the *value* of a reconstructive experience and practice for a fully trained and board-certified plastic surgeon performing cosmetic surgery. It's not that one field is more or less respected or regarded than the other, but that there is a perception that something is intrinsically different in the techniques, training, and demand of each. It's as if you can't be a stage actor if you are a television star or that you can't be a portrait artist if you are a house painter or that if you build new houses you can't renovate old ones. While this may be true for some, and perhaps the majority of such professions, it is not a truism for plastic surgery. The distinction is "real" in the public's perception, but artificial in many other respects. For some of the public, it is almost as if reconstructive work contaminates a cosmetic surgeon's artistic aura and cosmetic surgery's superficiality demeans a reconstructive surgeon's serious intent. The real question is: How important is reconstructive surgery experience in the performance of cosmetic surgery?

Because of its elective, cash-based, glamour-gilded allure, cosmetic surgery is a magnet for patients and doctors alike. No one has a trademark on the word "cosmetic," "cosmetic surgery," or "cosmetic surgeon." There isn't a stand-alone surgical residency devoted solely to cosmetic surgery (only fellowships following more extensive surgical residencies). Cosmetic surgery is a battleground for which individual doctors and professional societies vie. Plastic surgeons fear losing the war of public perception to organizations and individuals promoting themselves as cosmetic surgeons but who are not necessarily plastic surgeons. There are many societies and accreditation boards with the catchword "cosmetic" in their titles, none of which are formally recognized by the American Board of Medical Specialties that assists boards in developing and setting standards for physician certification in twenty-four different specialties.

Our very livelihood and survival as plastic surgeons depends on public perception. No one is battling to do hemorrhoid surgery. No one wants to be known as the colonoscopist to the stars. No one is advertising to the public the latest techniques in management of pressure sores, cleft lip repair, or orbital fractures. It was because of the public's misconception that "plastic and reconstructive surgeons" may not be as good at cosmetic surgery as "cosmetic surgeons" or may not even perform cosmetic work that led our major society of plastic surgeons (who are trained in all aspects of reconstructive and cosmetic surgery in an accredited surgical residency program) to vote a name change from the American Society of Plastic and Reconstructive Surgery (ASPRS) to the American Society of Plastic Surgeons (ASPS). While simplifying our name, it also served to de-emphasize, and effectively demote, reconstructive surgery, the unworthy stepchild.

This practical action, however well-intended, erased our historical roots and belied basic, irrefutable truths. One truth is that plastic surgeons *are* trained in reconstructive surgery. Not some of us—*all* of us. Second is that most cosmetic procedures and concepts have germinated and evolved from reconstructive experience. Third, it seems counterintuitive to think that a surgeon trained in reconstructive surgery, who has learned to manipulate the most fragile, traumatized, and abnormal of tissues in the most innovative ways, can't apply those same skills to manipulate healthy tissues that produce aesthetically pleasing results. Fourth is the fact that cosmetic surgery and reconstructive surgery are really part of a continuum and any division is because of the differences between patient and public perceptions, and not the surgeon or the task. Finally, what the public perceives as cosmetic surgery is, in fact, no different from reconstructive surgery but it just happens to be packaged in a way to give the effect of requiring a special talent.

This last point is exemplified in breast reduction surgery, where similar concepts and techniques may be thought of as reconstructive or cosmetic depending on the mindset of the patient and the coverage requirements of the insurance company, and not so much on the training or practice of the surgeon. Breast reduction is considered reconstructive if the breasts are so abnormally large or deformed as to produce unwanted physical side effects like skin rashes, ulcers, neck pain, or back pain. It is considered cosmetic if the surgery is done to enhance already normal breasts. To think that a reconstructive surgeon who operates on large breasts under an insurance policy is any more or less capable of producing an attractive breast than is a plastic surgeon who operates on that same breast outside of insurance coverage is simply false. Well-trained plastic surgeons strive both to produce the most attractive breasts for the patients while simultaneously relieving them of their symptoms. In fact, a surgeon who is able to wear both hats is preferable.

One case illustrates the extreme of this issue. A patient was sent to me from her gynecologist. She was a very pleasant, active woman in her sixties who had liquid silicone injected into her breasts thirty years ago as a then-accepted method of breast enlargement. This was a very common, but now illegal, procedure that produced quite natural and pleasing initial results but disastrous and deforming consequences years later; the liquid silicone formed hard nodules and lumps, migrated throughout the breast and chest, and even discolored, or, worse, extruded through, the skin. This patient had hard, painful lumps that discolored the skin of her breasts that, ironically, were now large, pendulous, and unattractive to her.

I recommended she undergo a modification of a reduction and lift operation whereby I would remove the majority of the silicone-impregnated breast tissue, shape the remaining skin, lift the nipple-areolar complex to a more normal and pleasing position, and place tissue expanders to make room for breast implants at a second operation. A general surgeon without any cosmetic surgery experience suggested a total mastectomy with removal of the nipple to get rid of all the silicone. A second plastic surgeon, looking for the most cosmetic result, advised a more limited breast reduction that preserved silicone impregnated glandular tissue, and the immediate placement of silicone gel implants. The patient eventually went with the latter surgeon because she was promised that the problem could be solved in one operation, not two. She came to me six months later, lamenting what I told her would be the consequence of her surgery: she had wonderful-looking breast, but had persistent painful nodules that required another operation—and perhaps a third or fourth until the majority of the offending silicone was removed.

Residency programs in plastic surgery predominantly concentrate on solving problems of function or deformity and in restoring normal anatomy. It is a time to learn basic techniques, familiarize oneself with anatomy, and make, correct, and analyze mistakes. Some programs are better at this than others and some are known for specific subspecialties such as free flap breast reconstruction, craniofacial and other pediatric surgery, or microsugery. Only recently have plastic surgery programs changed because one eye is on the post-residency environment, where it is getting more difficult to make a living performing solely insurance-reimbursed "medically necessary" reconstructive surgery and where competition is fierce for "non-medically necessary" cosmetic surgery. Where reputable plastic surgery residencies programs previously de-emphasized cosmetic surgery, significant experience in cosmetic surgery is now required within accredited programs and programs can be penalized for not having enough training in cosmetic procedures. Also, cosmetic or aesthetic surgery fellowships are now common so those surgeons who wish to forego the traditional route of spending their first five, ten, or fifteen years of practice performing predominantly reconstructive work before gravitating to cosmetic surgery can hit the ground running and claim special training. But this practice is really a result of an individual's interest, choices, and marketplace forces and not an intrinsic dichotomy of the field of plastic surgery.

The experience in reconstructive surgery, where solutions to problems are individualized and often unique, variations infinite, and creativity at a premium, presents a rich environment for the fertile, flexible, and innovative mind. Wartime bred whole subspecialities, such as cranio-maxillo-facial surgery, because of the myriad of wounds, functional as well as cosmetic. The advent of the motorized vehicle and industrial machines fostered new techniques of tissue mobilization such as muscle and fasciocutaneous flaps and new fields of replantation and microsurgery. In fact, some of the first limb replantation surgeries were performed in China prior to the Cultural Revolution because, rather than have society be burdened by non-productive citizens, replantation offered the possibility of returning productive workers into the fields and factories. Facial reconstruction for genetic and traumatic deformities gave birth to craniofacial surgery that ushered in an era of bony remodeling of the facial skeleton for cosmetic gain.

In my own experience, fixing facial fractures and learning craniofacial approaches made the endoscopic and subperiosteal face-lifting techniques that are all the rage that much easier and familiar. In Los Angeles, I co-founded a craniofacial clinic based on a multidisciplinary team treating patients with skull and facial skeletal deformities. I also performed calf implants in post-polio patients before applying it to a cosmetic patient. Learning from master cleft surgeon Dr. D. Ralph Millard, Jr. how to take apart a cleft lip and reconstruct it to look normal gave me a multi-dimensional understanding of the oral anatomy that makes lip enhancement a piece of cake. Moving around large regions of tissue to reconstruct missing or deformed areas of the torso gave me knowledge, experience, and courage in undertaking major body contouring and lifting procedures. Doing hundreds of breast reductions gives me a deeper feeling for the limits and contour requirements in manipulating the breast tissue for cosmetic effect. Correcting deformities of the eyelid with lid tightening and repositioning procedures and applying those principles to cosmetic eyelid procedures reduces the risk of complications in cosmetic patients, making for a safer and more anatomic operation. Having seen and solved problems gives me a healthy respect for the limits of tissue manipulation that undoubtedly assists in preventing complications. It also gives me confidence that if a problem develops, I can find a valid solution. It is not unlike having pilots with military experience fly commercial airliners or having people with inner-city experience become social workers. They've been there. Dentists doing facelifts and head and neck surgeons doing breast augmentations and gynecologists doing body-contouring procedures have not "been there." The same might be said for plastic surgeons coming straight out of residency and entering a practice of exclusively cosmetic surgery.

Many of the innovations and techniques in current use are direct descendants of the innovations and techniques found in reconstructive surgery. The real question is whether the surgeon is sensitive to the aesthetic desires of the patient. While the reconstructive surgeon's primary goal is to solve the functional or deformity problem, it does not mean that he or she will be happy with an "ugly" result; ugly may be the limitation of the situation. Good reconstructive surgeons will try to make their results as aesthetically pleasing as possible. It's just that their best results will usually fall short of normal and the patient's expectation is usually something less than that of perfection. So it is the patient, the problem, and the expectation that separate reconstructive from cosmetic, not necessarily the aptitude or attitude of the plastic surgeon.

One of the most satisfying compliments I received on more than one occasion was either a patient or another doctor remarking that I did "beautiful" reconstructive surgery. I pride myself in being meticulous with cleft lip surgery in the attempt to make a severely deformed face as normal and symmetric as possible. I look at a gaping wound and think about how to change its size, location, and even shape to produce the least conspicuous scar or deformity. Trying to build a nose from the basic building blocks of lining, cartilage, bone, and soft tissue challenges my technical skills and creativity far more than any "normal" rhinoplasty.

It is my belief and philosophy that cosmetic surgery and reconstructive surgery are really one and the same. When a face is abnormal because it met a windshield at sixty miles per hour or was unfortunate enough to be missing anatomical parts during in utero development, it is a reconstructive problem. When that same face is abnormal or undesirable (in the eyes of the individual) because it met the indomitable forces of aging or solar energy, it is a cosmetic problem. However, each situation presents a particular problem. Each problem requires an acceptable endpoint. Each problem requires some manipulation of anatomy to produce that desirable result. Each problem demands an individual solution that matches the expectation of the patient. Each problem has pitfalls and each solution risks side effects and complications. It is a simple matter of using all experience, knowledge, and techniques to move the patient from anatomical state A to anatomical state B. What caused them to get to point A in the first place may affect the solution, but it does not intrinsically make patients or the process of finding solutions any different.

I want my reconstructive results to be as attractive or normal as they can possibly be and I want my cosmetic results to be as renovating, functional, and natural as they can possibly be. The principles and even the techniques are the same. Both situations demand a natural, functional, and attractive surgery with the least amount of trauma, scar, side effect, and complication. The difference is not with me, the plastic surgeon, but with the patient and the problem... and perhaps the insurance plan. Problems are more tolerable when the perceived gain in reconstructive cases is large (i.e., when patients or body parts are so far removed from "normal"), but are less acceptable in cosmetic patients who may have less to gain because they are already "normal." Such was the rationale for allowing silicone gel implants for reconstructive use but not for cosmetic purposes during their recently ended fifteen-year moratorium. Protecting downside risk by minimizing complication is one of the major concerns in cosmetic surgery. All the experience surgeons have correcting deformities on all parts of the body allows them to know how to prevent many complications of cosmetic procedures and also to fix these complications when they do happen.

Lateral canthopexy to correct lid malposition is almost becoming routine in lower lid blepharoplasties. Managing problems associated with long, intersecting incisions in breast reduction, such as skin loss, delayed healing, or thick scars, led the way to modifications that eliminate more than half of the scars required for cosmetic breast lifts. Aggressive, deep degloving of the facial skeleton and transposition of soft tissue in facial reconstruction allows safe, quick, and maximal rejuvenation of the aging face. Open techniques in reconstructing and reshaping the cleft lip nasal deformity give rationale to cosmetic shaping of the nasal cartilage and bony structures. Acellular cadaveric skin (such as Alloderm) used to augment congenital and traumatic soft tissue depressions, atrophy, or other contour irregularities was my favorite material for aesthetic lip augmentation.

The contributions that reconstructive surgery has made to benefit cosmetic surgery go on and on. The complementary relationship between reconstructive and cosmetic surgery is even more evident in the thought process and analysis than in the technical execution. Cosmetic surgery is no different than reconstructive surgery except that the problems are less deforming, the solutions more restricted by what the patient will accept, and the margin of error less forgiving. Instead of being armed with standard cosmetic procedures that one applies to standard cosmetic complaints (i.e., sagging skin = facelift, tired eyes = blepharoplasty, nasal hump = rhinoplasty), it is more exact and correct to analyze the anatomical causes and relationships that give rise to these complaints from a structural and functional point of view, just as one would in trying to rebuild a nose or reconstruct a breast or change facial contours. In the end, it is really just *applied anatomy*. The face and body don't know if they ended up this way from trauma, the wrong genes, extreme weight loss, a series of pregnancies, the march of Father Time, or the cruelty of Mother Nature. After all, they're only bone, cartilage, fat, blood vessel, nerves, muscle, and skin.

There is no easy formula for determining the right surgeon for a particular cosmetic patient. It is as challenging at times as finding a capable and compatible mate. But excluding a surgeon because he or she does reconstructive surgery is not necessarily valid and one should judge a surgeon on the merits of his or her own cosmetic surgery experience and aesthetic sensitivity.

A good reconstructive surgeon often makes a great cosmetic surgeon. My own personal bias is that having a strong reconstructive background is a distinct advantage in performing cosmetic surgery and lacking that experience removes a valuable dimension and depth to one's knowledge and technical prowess.

CHAPTER 13:

THE MOST IMPORTANT THING ABOUT YOUR COSMETIC SURGEON IS…

"When I visit four plastic surgeons, why do I get five different opinions?"

—*A confused patient*

* * *

How long will a facelift last? What is the best way to do a breast reduction? How do we make someone beautiful? Is youth found in a bottle, a syringe, or with a scalpel? When should I have an eyelift? Is Botox better than Restylane? Is Restylane better than Juvederm? Are silicone implants safer than saline implants? Should I use implants, fat injections, thread lifts, or mid-facelifts to rejuvenate the cheeks? Can I do liposuction and a tummy tuck at the same time? Should I do surgery just when I start to age or should I wait until I look like I need it? Is it better to do a series of small procedures or one big one? Should teenagers have nose jobs? Do I have to have a browlift when I have an eyelift? How important is technique? How important is education? How important is experience? How important is it for your plastic surgeon to be famous?

Prospective patients seek answers to these endless questions. Countless television shows, newspaper stories, websites, and magazine articles explore these topics. I have personally answered well over a thousand questions like these on one interactive website alone. The questions are legitimate, reasonable, and can be answered in more than one way. Some might not have any answer at all. Nonetheless, each answer could be invaluable, even though it might be mere opinion. Each specific answer usually has a proponent and a critic. No answer is right and no answer is wrong. The public hungers for the truth and each media storyline or doctor, including me, may claim to have it. Confusion reigns.

If I were contemplating an eyelift (blepharoplasty), I would want to know if a laser or scalpel was better. If I were having a breast augmentation, I would want to know if I should place the implant above or below the muscle and whether to use saline or silicone gel implants. If I wanted body contouring, I would want to know if I should have the tummy tuck (abdominoplasty) prior to, after, or together with liposuction of the hips, flanks, and thighs, or not at all. In fact, why is there even an option? Why do some doctors do it one way and another a different way, and does that mean one of them is wrong? Before we consider plastic surgery, let's ask questions on another important topic on everybody's mind: no, not sex, but money.

One of the fundamental charges or goals an adult has in life is to earn a living. Earning a living is, by all intents and purposes, a necessity for the average, honest, unprivileged citizen. We need to earn income so that we can pay our bills, take care of our kids, feed, clothe, and house our families, help others less fortunate, and enjoy life as much as possible. Very few people can argue with that concept. Not doing these things is simply not an option. Hopefully, after the necessities are dispensed with, we'll have enough left over to start investing.

What to do with one's discretionary income, savings, or assets is a completely different matter than paying bills. Since discretionary income is, by definition, not absolutely necessary for the basic needs of living, it can be voluntarily placed in an infinite number of investment vehicles. Some investments are safe, predictable, and insured, like CDs, American Savings Bonds, and bank savings accounts. Some are risky, like oil and gas ventures, but promise bigger payoffs. Some involve stocks, from dividend-paying blue chips, to mid-caps, small-caps, and penny stocks. There are combinations of stocks grouped into funds, or baskets, or risk-based portfolios. There are real estate ventures and REITs, tax lien certificates, art and collectibles, franchises, commodities, bonds, partnerships, etc., etc., etc.

Everyone with disposable income faces the exact same question: *Where is the best place to invest my money?* The question is a basic and crucial one and the answer is, supposedly, basic and crucial as well. A right answer will provide financial security, peace of mind, an improved quality of life. Or so we hope. The wrong choice can produce financial disaster, an anxious future, and a diminished quality of life. Or so we fear. Everyone should want to know what the right answer is and how to avoid the wrong answer. A situation so elementary should have an obvious, straightforward, and uniform answer. Each investment vehicle mentioned has a legitimate and legal industry with real people working in these areas investing real money producing real, tangible, and measurable results. These are not schemes, fly-by-night ideas, or fraudulent endeavors. Why can't we get the real answer?

The answer to the elemental mathematical question, what is two plus two, exists. It doesn't matter who or where you are. Two plus two always equals four. Why doesn't a definitive answer to this elemental financial question exist, too? Isn't there a formula for financial success? What about answers to elemental cosmetic surgery questions? Someone should know.

Of course, if you go to a stockbroker, he will certainly recommend stocks. Buy if you feel stocks are going up and short them if you feel they are going down. If you talk to a real estate broker, she will recommend real estate. It's always a good time to sell when you are selling and it's always a good time to buy when you are buying no matter if the market is going up, down, or sideways. Within each profession, different people will recommend different types of products. Each broker will have a vested interest in what to recommend because that is what he or she is selling. He may be honest, but he is also biased. There is built-in conflict of interest.

A study by Chicago economist and co-author of *Freakonomics*, Steven Levitt, revealed a conflict of interest as evidenced by higher sales prices for brokers selling their own homes than those of their commission-paying clients. Priests have it. Rabbis have it. Politicians definitely have it. And doctors have it. Doctors don't intend for these conflicts of interest to affect their practice but often they do. They may be small, almost insignificant, but they're there. It is why many scientific studies, hospital appointments, and public presentations must be accompanied by a signed document revealing potential conflicts of interest. Doctors are human, too.

Non-financial conflicts of interest or biases are not necessarily bad or detrimental (although some definitely are). They are just products of experience, knowledge, or education. The line between bias and judgment is fine. Parents certainly are biased in their parenting. They have been affected by their own parents and rearing. Teachers are biased in their method of teaching. They have been influenced by educational theories and methods they have been taught or have experienced. Firefighters fighting fires might have more of a vested interest in preventing situations that promote fires so they recommend installing fire-retardant roofing. Special knowledge within one's field of interest can be beneficial in determining a more advantageous course of action. Obviously if doctors are intentionally distorting truth or their practice of medicine for their own betterment in a way that is injurious to the patient, that self-serving bias is not only morally suspect, but possibly criminal.

A recent study revealed that many doctors' recommendation of treatment is influenced by their own personal beliefs, whether cultural, social, or religious. In fact, doctors are not morally, ethically, or legally obligated to treat patients in a manner that may be contrary to their own personal beliefs. This is a major reason it is hard to find practitioners willing to inject a lethal dose of medication to carry out a legal death sentence. The same thing is true when doctors refuse to participate in abortions or provide for contraception education based on religious beliefs. Thus, this particular bias is actually assumed, accounted for, acceptable, and legally defensible. In other fields, this may actually be a good thing. That is, you would probably want a stockbroker to recommend stocks because he believes in them so much that he also invests in them personally. We want officers and directors of publicly traded companies to have a vested interest in the company by being stockholders. Women want spokespersons of a beauty company to actually use those products.

With doctors, we expect them to be unbiased and to look at illnesses or medical conditions from a purely scientific, not personal, point-of-view, so this revelation may be surprising to some. However, to some extent, specialization in medicine itself instills a bias toward or away from certain treatments. For example, a non-surgeon dermatologist may treat facial wrinkles with one method while plastic surgeons may treat them with another. Each will presumably favor his own specialty's bias and may influence a patient, however subtly, against the other specialty's approach. In obstetrics, it has been shown that physician factors and bias have contributed significantly to the increase in Caesarean sections.

Despite the usual assumption of the absence of bias and the predominance of objectivity, patients are themselves conflicted when it comes to subjectivity of answers. They don't necessarily just want the unfettered, unadulterated, cold, hard, statistical truth. Statistics are hard to digest and are often misleading, oversimplified, or overcomplicated and biased themselves. Statistical analysis is an incredibly complex field that I personally have never mastered and the distillation of data to produce a readily acceptable and understandable piece of usable information is often presented in a biased manner. In plastic surgery, a statistic like one type of facelift taking less time to perform, or being "less invasive" (a true oxymoron) than another may not admit the fact that it may also not last as long or produce as comprehensive or harmonious a change. Similarly, the fact that more patients wished they had gotten larger, rather than smaller, breast implants does not include the impression that those with implants that are too large are unhappier than those who are too small. This is presumably because they are unable to hide the excessive size while women who are a bit too small can simply choose a different bra. Stated data are often refuted by unstated data.

Patients prefer the reassurance of a real person making decisions. Patients often pose to the doctor the daunting question, "What if it were you? What if it was your sister wanting to get implants? What if you wanted a facelift? What if your brother wanted buttock implants? What would you recommend?" They might sincerely want to hear my personal bias in order to make a decision for themselves or they might actually hope to defer their decision entirely to me as their doctor, the keeper of their health and happiness, the arbiter of beauty. There is an expectation, even a demand, for the doctor's personal bias. They want to know. It is because the patients want to, and do, trust their doctors. Doctors are the accepted repository of medical knowledge and judgment. If it wasn't so, dispassionate computers would deliver medical care and patients wouldn't ask an opinion of someone they hardly know or don't respect or trust. The patient also expects that there is a correct answer to which the doctor is privy to or has an opinion about.

Science, statistics, medicine, physiology, anatomy, and material sciences, among other things, are crucial to the plastic surgeon's job. Just as financial advisors or brokers cannot do without financial data like revenue and earning statistics, economic forecasts, historical trends, cash flow statements, or price analysis, plastic surgeons cannot function without technical or statistical knowledge. But *how* we apply this knowledge, as I have tried to demonstrate, is dependent on the collaboration between cosmetic patient and plastic surgeon with the patient being the primary driver of the "treatment." Each patient brings his or her own set of values, beliefs, preferences, tastes, fears, and finances to the operating room. Many of these individual beliefs are the reason some people are sitting in the plastic surgeon's office in the first place and some are not. Some might feel that larger breasts are attractive and too large is not. But not all people feel that way. Some might believe that looking young helps attract the opposite sex. But not everyone else feels compelled to act on this belief. Some might believe that being able to wear certain clothes gives them enjoyment. Others may not place such value on this activity. So what does the surgeon, the other side of the equation, bring? How does a patient get what she wants with the surgeon she is with?

Each board-certified plastic surgeon has gone through years of formal schooling, accredited residencies, perhaps stints in research, and varying years of practical, hands-on experience. We read the same articles in the same journals. We have access to the same lectures and courses at the same professional meetings. While the science we learn is presumably the same and the statistical data we memorize is hopefully, but not always, relatively unbiased and unprejudiced, the application of that data and the experience of actual practice are probably, and often widely, different. A plastic surgeon fresh out of residency has a different perspective because of his training. He has different mentors and professors who instructed and influenced him. That same fresh-out-of-training surgeon has a different fund of knowledge than a surgeon in mid-career or one nearing retirement. It's not good or bad, or better or worse. It's just different.

When a patient meets a plastic surgeon, it doesn't matter who the patient is or who the plastic surgeon is, the goal at the end of the day is presumably to find some answers for that particular patient. Unless the patient is simply gathering information without having real intent on doing anything about it, like a high school student researching a project assignment, or she ends up bouncing back and forth between plastic surgeons in a Mobius strip of indecision like some do, something will and must be done: either she decides to do nothing or she decides to do something. To do nothing is still something, or, as the saying goes, "Not to decide is to decide." The questions then are "What is that something?" and "How is the decision made as to what that something is?" Your money has to go into some investment unless you hide it under a mattress or in some tin can (which can be a good decision in certain rare situations). But even if you do, there is a reason you choose to act this way. How do you justify your choices? How do doctors provide answers? How do you know whose answer to trust?

It bothered me when I asked a friend of mine why she kept fifty thousand dollars in a safety deposit box and she couldn't tell me why. If she had said her father lost all his money in the stock market crash or that banks were evil, capitalistic enterprises that take advantage of the poor and weak, I would have understood. But she didn't. She had no explanation or rationale for her actions. I suppose it was probably because she thought she might need the money and hadn't thought about what else to do with it. Doctors, on the other hand, should have a justification for everything they do.

What some patients don't realize is that the procedures and the techniques we have available are simply tools with which to accomplish a task. They are not the endpoints in themselves. They are not forever but transient until the next wave of change or improvement comes along. That is why this book is not about surgical techniques or "how-to's." Techniques get modified, become obsolete, or even vilified. They are oils on a palette, notes of a staff, words on a page, or investments in a portfolio. The procedures need to be employed in a certain manner to be useful. A patient coming in asking for liposuction is requesting a tool, not an endpoint. I will usually tell them to forget the liposuction. Just tell me what bothers you and what you will be happy with. Then we'll see if liposuction fits as an appropriate technique or tool. The technique needs to serve the goal. They are not the goals themselves.

Likewise, laser is not a procedure. It is a tool that can be good or bad, useful or not, safe or dangerous, depending on what type of laser is used in what situation at what energy setting for what purpose. A rhinoplasty is not a specific operation, nor is a facelift. A variety of tools and their application will comprise a specific rhinoplasty or facelift. One facelift is performed differently with different results than another facelift.

The endpoint is the desired change, not the procedure itself. Unfortunately, much of the information a patient receives outside the plastic surgeon's office is focused on technology, procedures, and tools, and not the most important aspect of being a cosmetic surgeon. If we look at all the injectable fillers that have propagated like field rabbits, we must wonder why we need over a hundred different materials. Like with all the investment vehicles, how does one choose? Why are there new ones coming into the marketplace?

Any good sports team, effective military mission, or successful business enterprise requires an operative strategy. There isn't only one strategy that is universally successful. Some teams like to overwhelm their opponent from the beginning while others prefer to wear them down over time. Stealth strategies in guerilla warfare are applicable in one situation, while "shock and awe" strategies may be appropriate in another. Some businesses believe in constant innovations while others rely on time-honored tradition and constancy. How do strategies get distinguished? Since plastic surgeons, theoretically, and to some extent practically, have the same tools, the same knowledge of anatomy, and the same data available from one office to the next, what will distinguish one plastic surgeon from another?

Each of the situations mentioned above has a strategy based on a set of principles. Those principles then encompass, and are derived from, a philosophy. Having a particular philosophy will set into motion a certain pattern of thinking that will produce a certain surgical strategy that then will impact a patient and what is done to that patient. As an extreme example—hopefully unfounded, although not entirely improbable—let's consider a philosophy that involves the belief that medical care is like any other business providing necessities of life: a food supplier, a clothing store, or an apartment building. It has making money as the primary motivating factor. A practice will then gear its behavior to maximize profits above all else. This philosophy got a lot of HMOs into trouble a decade ago. High-volume, low-cost, high-revenue, low-risk treatments will be de rigueur. Here, the cleft lip baby got thrown out with the bath water and many patients requiring costly treatment got left standing outside the front door.

In a different philosophy, a belief in using natural, biological, rather than alloplastic or synthetic, material will indicate certain techniques over others. Another philosophy might be to produce the most perfect result the patient wants regardless of the cost or magnitude of the techniques. Another common philosophy is voiced in "if it ain't broke, don't fix it."

The point is, surgical decisions, and medical practice in general, are governed by philosophies built on principles, one of which is immortalized in the Hippocratic Oath. These philosophies are individualized by practitioners as they travel through their careers and, yes, even in their personal lives. It is something that is not faced head-on or concretely in medical education and may not even exist in a doctor's consciousness. *But philosophy is, and should be, the most important factor in the treatment of patients*. A popular philosophy is to be cautious and conservative, a la Hippocrates, and to not accept new concepts until they are clinically proven to be beneficial (i.e., show me first). An opposing philosophy is to be aggressively proactive with new ideas and technology (i.e., I'd rather be too early than too late, first rather than last). Each philosophy will lead down a different path of decision-making and each decision on that path will be governed by the philosophy and a set of principles.

An extreme example is that of Chinese philosophy governed by Confucian concepts of filial piety. Here, the reverence towards one's ancestors is exemplified in preservation of one's body as an extension of those ancestors. Damaging, removing, or disrespecting one's body in the form of mutilation, amputation, or even physical enhancement through surgery (read "cosmetic surgery") may be taboo. Being philosophically pro-life or choice may determine a doctor's approach to abortion and birth control.

Without adhering to a certain philosophy or set of principles, surgical decision-making and opinion can become haphazard, even arbitrary. This does not mean one needs to be dogmatic, though treatment by rote is quite common. In fact, modern medicine's infatuation with standard protocols and practice parameters may mean a trend toward more automated treatment plans. However, a philosophy of flexibility in medical treatment is just as valid as a philosophy of rigidity. A philosophy celebrating customization and individualization is just as useful as a philosophy of standardization and protocol. In fact, one needs to be flexible in order to be creative. This concept is exemplified in the practice of surgical freehand called "cut-as-you-go." In retail, the philosophical road of "sell for less" leads to Wal-Mart while that of "the customer is always right" leads to Nordstrom's.

Between the rigid world of formulas, where answers are not dependent on who is solving the problem, and the chaotic world of arbitrary decision-making, where anything goes, lies the realm of subjective reasoning, where answers are very dependent on who is asked the questions. Decisions and actions in this world are definitely operator-based. How a surgeon views the world can impact his work just as bringing the task of painting a portrait to a realist or an impressionist will result in quite different works of art.

It is an insider's traditional belief that a surgeon's reputation, and this relates even more pointedly to cosmetic plastic surgeons, is based not so much on whom he or she operates, but on whom he or she doesn't; selectivity of patients and procedures is at least as crucial, if not more so, than doing the actual procedure "correctly." It will reveal the level of reasoning and judgment a doctor possesses. Liposuction is a prime example of this idea. Liposuction is simply a method to selectively remove fat through a small incision using a hollow cannula and a source of vacuum or other power. It is a basic and easy concept to grasp and not a very difficult mechanical maneuver to master. Yet applying it optimally in the optimal patient under the optimal circumstances is challenging. Since almost every person has fat, one needs an underlying philosophy to permit selectivity of application. How does one justify or not justify the use or non-use of liposuction when everyone has fat?

A surgeon motivated by an overriding philosophy of maximizing profits because cosmetic surgery is a business will act a certain way. One whose philosophy is to operate on only the most ideal candidate because it is a totally elective procedure will act another way. Another whose minimally invasive philosophy excludes large incision surgical treatments will make different recommendations. The decision-making goes beyond simple indications of use since not every one will be ideal or completely inappropriate. There are plenty of patients in the gray area of indications. *Just because you can* doesn't mean *you should* just as much as *just because you don't think you can* doesn't mean *don't try.*

It is not very satisfying to do a technically wonderful liposuction on the wrong kind of patient in the wrong clinical situation. That might be just as egregious as doing a poor liposuction on an ideal patient in an ideal clinical situation. Whether a doctor uses ultrasonic liposuction, laser liposuction, or vacuum liposuction is probably less important than how a doctor assesses a patient. Having a rationale for saying "no" or "not now" to a patient may be a far better tool than the latest technological advance. (My standard of a 'healthy, stable lifestyle' is a direct result of my philosophy of 'cosmetic surgery is unnecessary').

Because plastic surgery finds itself in a media-sensitive world, especially here in Beverly Hills, often the opposite situation applies. That is, plastic surgeons are judged by who ends up in their office and whom they reportedly, correctly or not, operated on. Operating on a big-name celebrity can add luster to one's name while the more prudent and wise act of turning down a celebrity may not register at all in the public's opinion. Yet the latter may say more about a surgeon, his judgment, and how good of a doctor he is. Fame is not a reliable gauge of quality.

It used to be that plastic surgeons most commonly received patient referrals through word of mouth—either satisfied patients or physician colleagues—or by reputation, well-deserved or not. But now in the Google and E! Entertainment environment of instant information and publicity, potential patients can bypass these traditional sources and find almost anything about a doctor: his education, his credentials, his licensures, his malpractice history, photos of his past patients. What is not readily accessible in this gigabyte world is information about *how* he thinks and *why* he thinks the way he thinks. Did he become a doctor because he revered the caring treatment his medical father rendered or because his medical father never made any real money and now he wants to avenge his poverty? Is he by nature cautious or a risk-taker?

In reality, I have never had a patient ask me in a direct way, "What is your philosophy on plastic surgery?" or "What is your philosophical take on breast implants?" Perhaps it means that they already know what my philosophy is. But more than likely, it is because philosophy is not what is on her mind when coming to see a plastic surgeon about a facelift, a breast augmentation, or even liposuction. I often wondered what a colleague of mine would say if these questions were posed to him or her. He might stare at me with a vacuous look. Few people want to talk in abstract, flowery language about a grand scheme of man's, or woman's, purpose on earth. They don't want to hear me (or any other plastic surgeon) wax eloquently and critically on the intricacies of decision-making in plastic surgery. They want to know what they will look like after their facelift, how much the breast augmentation will cost, and when they can start exercising after they've been suctioned. Philosophy is about as far from their mind as how my favorite baseball team, the Boston Red Sox, is going to affect my conversation with them.

Yet, when we look at how humans live their lives, how they invest their disposable income, what they are willing to die for, and how they make choices, it is all dependent on a particular and individual philosophy, or lack thereof, whether they are cognizant of it or not. Life is not entirely random. Decisions are not haphazard but occasionally might just seem so. That is why we have Republicans and Democrats, religious fanatics and atheists, liberals and conservatives, socialists and capitalists, conservationists and consumerists, hawks and doves, etc., etc., etc. People polarize themselves in contrasting philosophical camps. We are not innately different. We just have different values and beliefs.

Similarly, how a plastic surgeon makes his decision, how he answers questions, and how he performs a particular procedure will, in large part, be based on his own philosophy. We *must* have a philosophy about what we are doing. Answers should not be given solely by rote. Plastic surgeons should have a structure within which they are able to value ideas and actions. We need a set of principles, both surgical, as perhaps set forth by my mentor, Dr. D.Ralph Millard, Jr., and his mentor, Sir Harold Gillies, as well as non-surgical, by which we justify our judgment. Without these, we are like children without a moral, ethical, legal, intellectual, or religious foundation whose compass of decision-making is uncalibrated, unfocused, and uncentered and whose conversations are mere regurgitations or mimicry of what they have heard. Facts, data, techniques, opinions are all floating around in our plastic surgical universe cluttering our thinking until they can be collated and organized into a cohesive plea for one or another course of action. To do this, one needs a philosophy.

Choosing the *right* philosophy is less of the issue than choosing *a* philosophy. We chose a philosophy and then the patient can chose us. Philosophies are not right or wrong. They cannot be proved better or worse. They are central beliefs that support other beliefs and they shape our course of action. And like the second law of thermodynamics dealing with entropy, it takes input of energy to create order out of chaos. Random decision-making takes no effort. You can simply flip a coin or spin a dial. Rationalized and orderly decision-making requires much effort.

Patients can select out a doctor whose philosophy is not compatible with theirs. If a patient is leaving decisions entirely in the hands of her surgeon, what that plastic surgeon's philosophy is could be the most important thing to know. If the plastic surgeon doesn't have one, you might ask yourself how this surgeon will make the decisions he will be making and why he answers the questions the way he does. That, along with his personality traits, will often influence how he performs surgery in the operating room.

All this becomes starkly apparent when I supervise residents in plastic surgery and observe them trying to discuss what they are going to do with prospective patients. Most residents have not had the time or experience or background to develop a philosophical approach to their work. They are truly "in training." Many will never develop a cohesive philosophy in their career because they have not been oriented to the value and necessity of having one. They struggle with analyzing patients, understanding the anatomy, learning the options, and making choices. Often they make decisions without knowing why they are making a particular decision and why that decision is favored over another. They often agonize over minute trivialities like what sutures to use, whether a new technique is any good, or where to put scars. They lose sight of the reason they are even in the room with their patient to begin with.

As I have said elsewhere, the relationship and trust between doctor and patient in practice is not unlike that between spouses in marriage. Ideally, you wouldn't trust your spousal life with someone with whom you didn't agree or share common goals (although many people actually do). It's hard enough when you do agree. Why would you trust your face and body, or life, to a plastic surgeon whose philosophy didn't exist or one you didn't accept, understand, or feel was compatible with your own?

CHAPTER 14:

WHY COSMETIC SURGERY IS SOOOOOO EXPENSIVE...OR NOT

Question: What is the scientific name for cosmetic surgery?

Answer: A wallet biopsy.

Question: If liposuction were a game show, what would it be called?

Answer: *Sucking for Dollars.*

* * *

As crude as it may seem, cosmetic surgery is as much about the business of making money as it is about the art of making patients beautiful. It is a truism that the business of beauty is not altruistic; if the ability to turn a profit were erased, cosmetic surgeons would evaporate like the morning fog in Santa Monica Bay. Sure, we love what we do and we take pride in the surgical result and the joy it brings to our patient. But we don't practice cosmetic surgery as a hobby and much of what is happening in plastic surgery is due to the shift of income away from reconstructive surgery. While it is not solely about business, patients understand and generally accept that there is a business side to our profession.

At some point in a conversation about cosmetic surgery, someone will raise the question of cost. Not uncommonly, it is the first and only question asked during the initial phone call to the doctor's office. Quoting a price sight unseen is usually discouraged since it presumes, among other things, that the patient's idea of what he or she wants is appropriate, that the procedure he or she is thinking about is the same procedure for which the quote is given, and that the procedure named is uniformly executed by all surgeons, none of which may be true. Nonetheless, many plastic surgeons' offices provide quotes, or at least estimates, with enough wiggle room to modify in case the assumptions are incorrect.

There is an art to quoting fees over the phone. The plastic surgeon wants to get you into the office for the initial consultation; he certainly doesn't want to scare you off. But he can't commit to a particular procedure without fully evaluating you, including your ability to pay. A patient also doesn't want to waste her time if she can't afford the surgery, although some will see us just out of curiosity. Consultants advising plastic surgeons in this art are also interested in techniques that convert phone inquiries into office appointments while quickly screening out patients who will squander the doctor's precious time. Through the years, as cosmetic surgery as a business has evolved and matured, a whole cottage industry has emerged to assist employees in a doctor's office with this delicate task of phone etiquette and financial consultation. Not surprisingly, a surgical consultant whose sole duty is to match the patient with a procedure and a price is often the highest-paid employee in the office. As possibly the most important employee in a plastic surgeon's office, she is coached in the delicate art of "the sell."

Advertisement may use fee quotes as teasers with disclaimers in miniscule print at the bottom of the page, excluding items like anesthesia, operating room charges, implants, or follow-up appointments. They may simply refer to the uninformative phrase "starting at." Professional societies advise against quoting fees prior to interviewing and examining a patient but, in the end, the "humanistic calling" of being a physician and healer of men and women has to be reconciled with the "fiscal responsibility" of cosmetic surgery as a livelihood. This business is not much different than any other business offering luxury goods; sometimes the necessity of just getting the customer into the office wins out.

My particular practice is to not discuss fees before I have appropriately evaluated the patient. In fact, I may not even quote fees after the initial consultation. This may put me at a disadvantage because many patients (perhaps 30 percent) may be influenced primarily by price and they can't understand why I don't have a set price for a facelift or breast reduction or rhinoplasty. My philosophy of customization and individual planning does not lend itself to accurate, generic price quotes. Even a "simple" request for a breast augmentation may not take into consideration the different prices in implants or different operating times for various techniques on different types of patients with different types of breasts. A patient may benefit from a small lift or even a combination of reduction, lift, and augmentation to achieve the desired result but not consider this when calling about a "simple boob job." They may have constricted or tuberous breasts, requiring more extensive surgery. Large implants placed in small, flat breasts with chest wall asymmetry may require more or less dissection and operating time than small implants in fuller breasts.

These variables cannot be adequately or honestly evaluated without talking to and examining the patient. Asking how much a "breast job" or facelift costs is like asking how much a kitchen costs. It depends on what kind of kitchen you want and how much work you put into building it. Often you won't know until you have met with the designer a number of times. The time and effort in planning the operation cannot be forgotten in the overall cost; custom art or manufacturing is typically more expensive than reproductive art or mass production.

Patients come from all walks of life. They have varying degrees of financial ability to pay, different levels of desire for cosmetic surgery, and wildly disparate expectations of costs. Some patients look for the lowest price like shopping online for airline tickets or vacation packages. Others expect, and want, to pay more for excess pampering and celebrity treatment, avoiding the factory-line practices. There may be a belief that if you are too inexpensive, you can't be good or, conversely, if you are the most expensive, you must be the best.

Local competition plays a role and even the location itself can be a factor. People expect to pay more for a procedure in Beverly Hills than in Tarzana or El Monte. Being in an office in a specific, premier building on a more "fashionable" street may command a premium; have you ever heard of Fourth Avenue plastic surgeons? Some want to pay more because they pride themselves in knowing they can buy at Tiffany's or Gucci's and not have to go to Target or K-Mart (no offense to any of these retailers).

To demonstrate the contradiction inherent in perception, one patient may indignantly ask why one surgeon is twice as expensive as another while a different patient may be suspicious as to why that same second surgeon is only half as cheap as the first. Yet as in most businesses, there is no substitute for pleasant personalities, impeccable reputations, and prompt, courteous, personalized service.

Some doctors will resort to discounts that may be a kind of lost leader lure or may be quite legitimate, as in the case of professional courtesy, hardship cases, or multiple, repeat, or volume business. Some prices are determined predominantly by costs found in cost-plus systems where a certain profit is added to the cost of delivering the service. This is common in construction contracting where a profit margin is added to the cost of materials and labor, or in fees for injectables like Botox or fillers where the cost of treatment is quoted as dollars per unit of Botox or dollars per cc's or syringes of filler.

Some plastic surgeons look at cosmetic surgery as the purest form of free market; the competitive, capitalistic market will determine the price based on supply and demand. Their goal, like any respectable capitalistic enterprise, is to maximize the profit. Each patient has complete freedom in determining how much a treatment is worth to her. In that scenario, assuming information is complete and accurate, no one will overpay for surgery. No matter the variations, the reason that cosmetic surgery prices are legitimate is that cosmetic surgery is inherently unnecessary.

Each patient can freely choose to refuse to undergo the elective surgery since there is no risk to not undergoing these procedures in the first place. It is probably the one and only place in medicine where true free market forces prevail. There is no third party, like the federal government in the case of Medicare, the state government in the case of Medicaid, or insurance companies in the case of reconstructive surgery, interfering with or controlling prices. No one is going to be arrested for asking thousands of dollars for a Louis Vuitton bag or a Harry Winston necklace, unless they are knockoffs. The patient/client may, at any time, just walk away or go down the street. Conversely, no one will be underpaying for the surgery since the surgeon is never obligated to perform an elective procedure; he can always say no.

The motivations for physicians in pricing their services are not uniform. Some go by market price, taking a middle road so as to be competitive with the majority of other doctors. Others trade price for increased volume and others feel they are inherently "better" or have some educational, service, celebrity, notoriety, or location premium to justify being "the most expensive act in town." Younger surgeons just starting out in practice may have a strict business philosophy of never losing a customer. A dollar in your pocket is still a dollar in your pocket and you never want to lose a patient to your competition—unless it's a "problem" patient. These doctors may bargain with a patient to lower the price in order to ensure performing the procedure and not lose a potential source of income. As long as you are straightforward with the patient, there is no single right way to price procedures. As in beauty itself, expensiveness is relative in the eye of the beholder.

The third-party payer system in health care is in direct contrast to this unique situation where supply and demand, not preferred provider or HMO contracts or Medicare politics, determine cost. With insurance companies or the government as fiduciary intermediary, the marketplace is disrupted for the goal of providing healthcare services for an ever-increasing population of eligible enrollees. By pooling resources (taxes and premiums), sharing risks, budgeting services, and standardizing prices, these programs provide services to citizens who can't afford them individually (i.e., most of us). Healthcare providers, whether they are facilities like hospitals and labs, or people like physicians and therapists, must decide if they want to play or not play within these systems. Most will choose to play because they need the volume of patients until the reimbursement becomes so low that enough people can afford to and are willing to pay more to go outside the system. Some states, like Massachusetts, threaten to distort the marketplace directly by obligating physician participation in the Medicare entitlement program.

In addition, the pricing of procedures is often in direct contradiction to marketing theory where increasing demand usually means increasing prices. Instead, in order to adhere to a "near-zero sum" policy, a popular procedure in high use may eventually cause a *reduction* in price rather than the expected increase in price due to high demand. This is what happens in Medicare where reimbursement can be cut when a procedure is over-utilized. In fact, over the last couple of decades, the future solvency of Medicare has come under question. It has evolved from a social safety net to a legal entitlement. Insurance companies, in the form of HMOs and PPOs, have increased their clout and their obligations to shareholders. In the meantime, Medicare fees have gone from being an effective floor on prices to a calculated ceiling.

Cosmetic surgery still remains an un-benefited product that patients pay for out of their own pockets. In third-party payer systems, the patients don't see the real price of a covered service but only the co-payment, perhaps 10 or 20 percent. This can lead to overuse of services since patients are effectively paying for only a small percentage of the actual price. It is like getting an automatic, built-in discount. Of course consumers might still feel they are paying too much if they believe medical care should be a universal benefit or that medical insurance should insure them against any and all costs of medical treatment. With cosmetic surgery, the patient (or maybe the spouse/uncle/parent/ boyfriend/girlfriend) sees every dollar of cost. Surgeons, on the other side, can determine for themselves what fee they are willing to work for and, for the most part as sole practitioners, are knowledgeable of their cost basis. If they are the only act in town, they can demand higher fees. In a competitive environment, fees are held in check and individualized by perception or demonstration of varying quality of outcome.

Quality is a key element in any marketplace, whether perceived or real. Advertising is largely designed to attempt to produce a perceived superiority, or to bring to the public's awareness true and measurable differences in quality, cost, products, or services. The fact that cosmetic surgery is performed by individual doctors on individual patients using different techniques and different products underscores the fact that *not all procedures are the same.* That is, a facelift with one doctor may not be the same as a facelift with another. A liposuction procedure on one patient may not amount to the same procedure on a similar patient. One cheek implant may be quite unlike another cheek implant. Thus you can't really compare prices like you would two identical forty-two-inch Sony plasma televisions, one from Best Buy and another from Sears.

The third-party payer system has evolved to where there are major influences on the cosmetic surgery marketplace. Because it is impossible for *all* plastic surgeons to earn a *desired* standard of living performing *only* third-party payer-reimbursable reconstructive surgery, cosmetic surgery is a natural outlet. Medical economics is effectively a zero-sum game with a finite amount of federal and private dollars allocated to all projected medical claims. Doctors, hospitals, and laboratories providing medical care, and the pockets of company executives and shareholders compete for healthcare funding in the private sector. Some doctors will supplement their income with cosmetic procedures or look to transition into cosmetic surgery, or decide to forego reconstructive surgery altogether.

The general trend of doctors entering the cosmetic surgery field will tend to put downward pressure on prices, especially in highly competitive places. Recent statistics show that as the number of cosmetic procedures is increasing in the United States, especially for minimally invasive or non-surgical procedures like injectables, the volume of reconstructive procedures reimbursed by insurance is decreasing. However, there are also factors that will tend to inflate prices.

Doctors who are doing reconstructive surgery may have a "rob Peter to pay Paul" philosophy. That is, take from the rich so that the poor can get necessary treatment. As revenue from reconstructive surgery diminishes due to less volume and less reimbursement per case, doctors look to cosmetic surgery to make up the shortfall. With the resultant enlarging supply of providers of cosmetic surgery, each doctor's volume will be diluted out especially in an area that attracts plastic surgeons. This is certainly true for the "mecca" of plastic surgery, Beverly Hills, a small town with a permanent population of only around thirty-five thousand. Here, doctors performing cosmetic procedures are as plentiful as hairstylists and gardeners with nearly seventy board-certified or board-eligible plastic surgeons with practices in the Beverly Hills Triangle—an area of less than one square mile—resulting in a per capita ratio of one surgeon per five hundred residents! Since fixed costs of running a surgical practice (i.e., rent, personnel, supplies, insurance, continuing medical education dues) continue to go up, doctors will tend to try to raise fees to make up for lower volume and thus counteract the downward pressure on fees caused by increased competition. Cosmetic surgery, being a luxury item of sorts, provides justification for being the most expensive game in town. The rich flock to buy the most expensive cars, watches, jewelry, and houses. In cosmetic surgery, patients are suspicious of the lowest cost provider and few respectable doctors want to be known as the cheapest act in town.

One example of the recent trends affecting plastic surgeons is the presence of panel discussions at national meetings where plastic surgeons explore the fiscal challenges of running a practice specializing in breast reconstruction, a highly necessary, complex, legally mandated, but poorly reimbursed process. The same has been true for reconstruction of congenital deformities such as craniosynostosis and cleft lip and palate.

With the trend out of reconstructive surgery and into cosmetic surgery, a resultant irony is that the cost to augment normal breasts is more than the reimbursement to reconstruct a post-mastectomy deformity. Medicare will pay about four hundred dollars to do an implant reconstruction of the breast while a cosmetic augmentation costs many times that. The reimbursement to plump up a normal lip exceeds the reimbursement to reconstruct a cleft lip. It is perhaps counterintuitive to think that one can justify being paid handsomely for assuming the anxiety and risk of performing unnecessary, but highly desirable, surgery on normal, healthy patients but not expect to be rewarded for saving a patient's life or limb. But that is the contrarian world in America, where recreation and pleasure often out-trumps the necessities of life. I make no apologies for this upside down world since it is not of the doctors' doing. It's just the way things are and it does allow some surgeons who like to do reconstruction to continue to do it (or is it that it *requires* them to do the financially more-rewarding cosmetic surgery?).

During the medical insurance crisis of the early 1990s that drove the first half of the Clinton presidency, I had idealistically thought plastic surgeons were the perfect specialty to help save the system since we were the ones who could afford to subsidize the under-insured patient population because we had cosmetic surgery to pay our bills. Very few other medical specialties had that luxury.

I suppose from a purely business point of view, elective cosmetic surgery can be priced at whatever the market will bear. Every potential patient has his or her own level of desire, motivation, and financial wherewithal as much as each surgeon has his or her own expense obligations and own desire and motivation for work, income, and quality of life (i.e., children, dependents, expensive hobbies, and ex-spouses).

If one looks at cosmetic surgery as art—which I think is valid—one only has to market a procedure to a single individual. What that individual is willing to pay determines the price. It is not necessarily a mass-market situation. The inherent assumption is that the patient is able to get what he thinks he wants in terms of the result before the art is actually done. The surgery then becomes a piece of commissioned artwork. The real risk of the business goes beyond the medical risks of the surgery: either the patient doesn't get what he wants, doesn't like what he gets, or gets a complication that places additional financial obligation or psycho-emotional burden on patient and doctor.

In the end, a major driving force in justifying higher rather than lower prices is that surgeons are compensating themselves for taking on *the risk, anxiety, and responsibility of operating on normal, healthy people.* It is the management and the assuming of downside risk that fuels the feeling that doctors need to be reimbursed for the stress and strain of operating on normal, healthy human beings. It is daunting to feel that you might make very, very sick every patient who is basically, and in reality, not sick at all.

In continuing medical education courses and symposia on complications of cosmetic procedures, devastating outcomes that can literally happen to any

healthy patient or well-intended, well-trained doctor can make our blood freeze. Gory and tragic pictures of debilitation and deformity from liposuction,
facelifts, and breast surgery force me to give serious
consideration to foregoing elective cosmetic surgery
or changing professions entirely; there must be an
easier way of making a living. Well-placed patients,
whether they are celebrities, socialites, well-connected
housewives, or busy aestheticians or trainers—all normal, functioning, productive people—can as much
enhance your practice when things go right or destroy
it when things go wrong. One well-known surgeon
went so far as to say that early on in his career he
looked at patients as being afraid of him, while later
he looked at patients as potential liabilities that *he*
should be afraid of. Some doctors had patients who
rented billboards condemning them after a surgery
gone bad. Some had picketers decrying their skills
on sidewalks in front of their offices; in fact, there are
three marching right now outside a plastic surgeon's
building.

The popularity of the Internet and social networks
has given rise to websites devoted to bad-mouthing a
doctor. Some are merely scam sites designed to extort
money from doctors petrified at the thought of losing their hard-earned reputations overnight. More
than a few plastic surgeons have been murdered by
dissatisfied patients or their loved ones. Some doctors,
notably during the silicone gel implant crisis of the
early 1990s, entered bankruptcy because of malpractice suits brought on by disgruntled patients, aggressive lawyers, and a suspicious public environment. All
this pressure has gotten to a number of plastic surgeons who decided to commit suicide. There are few

professions where one false turn can cost you your home, savings, career, and even life. And all this perhaps from a mere perception of injury or harm; ugliness and failure are in the eye of the beholder.

In some ways, plastic surgeons performing elective cosmetic surgery are like "closers" in baseball. Closers are relief pitchers brought into the game at the end to protect the lead and preserve a win. They are some of the most highly paid pitchers per pitch thrown, namely because they can only lose, not win (unless they first lose the lead). *They are compensated handsomely to not lose.* Their entire day's wages can hinge on a single pitch.

Of course, expensiveness or inexpensiveness is relative. I have had patients ask why a procedure is so expensive and others ask why that same procedure is so reasonable. It also depends on that patient's past experience. If they've had a facelift for fifty thousand dollars, they think my fee is reasonable. But if they've never had a one-hundred-and-fifty-dollar facial, they might think my price is outrageous. They might compare the price of cosmetic surgery with the price of a new luxury car and think they are getting a bargain, while measured against the cost of higher education, they might think it is a waste of money.

Money can always color perceptions and influence actions. I always ask the prospective patient not to think about money or finances when they come in. I suggest they pretend they have all the money in the world, which some seem to have, or that they are flat broke, which, surprisingly and strangely enough, some are. The first goal is to determine and define what they want and the second is to decide on what I need to do to help them achieve their goals. Once that purity of psycho-emotional well-being, anatomical analysis, and plastic surgical technology is understood, respected, and adhered to, then I can haggle over the fees if I want. There is nothing to say that I shouldn't make as much profit as I can or that I can't practically give away procedures if I want to as long as I am not blatantly discriminatory or violating an illegal or ethical quid pro quo (for example, exchanging free surgery for free publicity). *There is wide latitude in pricing for individual cosmetic patients.*

Some doctors may do surgery on a celebrity for next to nothing, hoping any publicity will bring additional business. They might even make deals if the celebrity agrees to talk to the press about their surgery. Others may charge celebrities more because of the added risk they represent and added care they might demand. The important point is to perform the procedural steps that will provide the patient with the highest degree of satisfaction no matter who they are or what they are paying. It does no good to perform a procedure that the patient can afford but does not produce the intended result, just as it may be unsatisfying to turn away a good, and potentially extremely grateful, patient who can benefit from surgery just because you cannot maximize profitability.

The ideal situation is to have both the patient and the doctor believe that the end result of the surgical treatment can be a reasonable and satisfying investment. I tell patients they have to be comfortable with *all* aspects of the surgery: surgeon, anesthesia, procedure, facility, explanations, risks, *and* price. Discomfort with any of these components may hinder an optimal result. In the end, patients should never feel forced to do anything with which they are not comfortable. They must be guilt-free.

The interesting thing about art is that price has absolutely nothing to do with raw materials. A value of a painting is not contingent on how much an artist paid for his canvas or oils. Conversely, a sculptor can sink a lot of money into a hunk of marble or bronze and end up with just a hunk of marble or bronze. The same can be said about cosmetic surgery. Certainly there is a bottom line because there are real costs to consider. Just to have someone walk into the office is an expense and to actually put them to sleep and operate on them generates costs. But the real price goes beyond real costs. It includes the tangible cost and the opportunity cost of years of post-graduate education, the cost of fear of failure, the profit of a successful outcome in terms of future referrals, the cost of stress and anxiety that one might offend the Hippocratic Oath and do some harm. It also factors in, to some extent, the elusive benefit that an individual patient will receive from the procedure. I never minimize the motivation behind each patient who is so willing to lay down his or her body for us and to tempt the forces of nature and tease the spirit of Narcissus. We should never underestimate the inherent value of intrinsic trust.

One also has to remember that once a surgeon has operated on a patient, that patient is his or hers until they "divorce," a rare but often painful and potentially expensive experience. That means that every little concern, every day following the operation, every thought a patient has about the treatment, is the surgeon's responsibility.

This is true of all professionals. What compounds the importance is that, once again, cosmetic patients have nothing "wrong" with them to begin with. They are anatomically and functionally normal people seeking an improvement in the quality, not quantity, of life. Any setback, imperfection, complication, anxiety, dissatisfaction, or financial strain on the patient will be measured against his or her world *without* those problems. If enough surgeries are done, some of these problems are going to arise. That is the nature of surgery. No money in the world can compensate the honorable doctor or healthy patient for that unfortunate end result. For that reason alone, cosmetic plastic surgery is expensive. Being unable to return art is no joke.

CHAPTER 15:

PUTTING IT ALL
TOGETHER...MY WAY

* * *

Accompanying every story is a backstory. In a good novel or movie, it is an essential element that drives the plot and characters. In the blockbuster film *Star Wars*, the backstory surrounding Luke Skywalker became the subject of an entire trilogy of prequels relating the story of his father, Anakin, and how Anakin fell to the dark side to emerge as Darth Vadar. So it is with my patients and why they are sitting in my office seeking plastic surgery. I may not go back four generations into their family history, but I am just as interested in their backstory as in the actual surgery requested and I will spend a fair amount of time investigating it.

"Just talk to me," I encourage them. Mull it over. Agonize over it. Be embarrassed. But get it out. Patients should be willing, if not eager, to share their story. The passive, reticent patient dutifully listening to the pontificating plastic surgeon doesn't work for me.

I want to know the process by which a patient ends up in my office revealing her intimate details and fears to a stranger and inviting surgical invasion of her body. How long has she been thinking about this? When did she decide to make an appointment? Why did she decide to make the appointment? Why now and not before? Who corroborates, objects to, or encourages her in her concerns? What are her relationships and what do those people know or think about her consultation? How secure is she in her relationship? How secure is she in her job? What was her relationship with her parents or siblings? Each person's life is a journey and I want to understand that journey. All of this familiarizes me with the patient as a human being, the very beginning of the fifth dimension and the heart of plastic surgery as art. I operate on people, not body parts.

At first, as I consult with the patient, I mostly listen. Psychiatrists practice their craft by listening—so, too, good parents. And good orchestral conductors. And good teachers. And good executives. I let the patient lead me to where she wants to go. I want to hear how she conceptualizes her situation and how she expresses herself. I try to avoid suggestion. I force her by my silence to show me things from her unique point of view. I suppress my personal beliefs, feelings, and opinions. Too often I have seen surgeons lead patients down a path, making presumptions and drawing conclusions that are less about the patient than about the surgeon. While the surgeon must have an ego, *cosmetic plastic surgery is about the patient's ego, not the surgeon's.*

Even as the patient presses me for my opinion, I actually tell her that what I like isn't important; it's what *she* likes or doesn't like that is crucial. She will indicate how deeply a problem may affect her. She will reveal her expectations and her fears. While this may initially seem distant from her immediate surgical concerns, in this way I can begin to gauge the risks and visualize the benefits.

In seeking her own truths, I will pressure her to be specific. At times I am sure I sound like an idiot, or a nag, or an arrogant intellectual. What do you mean by attractive? Nice? Natural? Better? What specifically are you referring to when you say "here," "this," "that," or "in general"? Are you talking about the fold or the crease below the fold? The texture or the contour? The way it looks or the way it feels? How much is too much? Are you looking at an anatomical structure but talking about an emotional effect? Will the structural change lead to such an effect? Is perception of a change just as good as actual physical change? Do you want the nose to really be smaller or just to look smaller? Is the nose truly small, just proportionally small, or only perceptively small? It will be hard, tedious, and exasperating work and, at times, I admit I might sound like President Clinton trying to define the word "is." But you can't hit the target unless you define the target.

The goal for me is to understand the patient as a psycho-emotional human being with a three-dimensional anatomy in order to place her at what I refer to as point A. Point A is who she is at this place and time in my office. The backstory is important because it gives a setting to judge how or if point A is moving or will move and what the journey was to get her to this point (i.e., the fourth dimension). Remember that the optimal time to assess a patient is when she achieves a healthy, stable lifestyle. The stable part can only be determined over the dimension of time. If a person weighs two hundred and twenty, I want to know if he came from two hundred and forty or one hundred and eighty, and over what period of time, whether in a straight line or circuitous path, and how fast. If a person claims she has aged, I want to know how she has aged. Examination of past photos from her younger days can be telltale. If she says something has affected her, is it getting better or worse and how quickly? The medical objectivity I bring to their situation must be reconciled with the subjectivity of their personal point-of-view.

Critical to this initial assessment are standard photographs. Having looked at all of my patients through these photographs, it is the method by which analysis can be calibrated. My patient and I can see the exact same image from the exact same perspective. I will rarely produce a recommendation or even an assessment of the problem, and certainly not a surgical fee quote, without first taking and examining these photographs.

Once I have established my patient at point A and have determined that she is in a healthy, stable lifestyle, defining what our goal (i.e., Point B) is will be the next challenge. Visual aids, previous examples, photographs, drawings, and just plain verbal discourse will help paint a clearer picture. *Collaboration is the ideal working relationship.* This picture requires a balance between specificity in anatomy and flexibility in expectation. The search for precision is measured against a theoretical margin of error. Predictability persistently battles unpredictability. Perfection is strived for but rarely obtained and never guaranteed.

The first consultation is a general airing out session when my prospective patient describes the reasons and circumstances of why she is in my office. While she is providing the history to me, she will also get an anatomy lesson based on my examination that will explain why she is seeing what she is seeing. The more she grasps the anatomical basis of her problem, the more rational the anatomical treatment will seem. A general complaint or anatomical condition (i.e., loose neck or sagging breasts) should not automatically dictate a generic procedure (i.e., necklift or mastopexy). Rather, each *component* of the complaint should be anatomically accounted for in a *customized* solution. I will also explain my philosophy and approach to her, orienting her as to how decision-making will proceed and what input I might expect of her as collaborator. She cannot be a passive bystander in the reshaping of her life.

My patient leaves my office after the first visit not uncommonly in a state of confusion, having been flooded with lessons in anatomy, physiology, and philosophy without a clear recommendation or price in hand. This may be unsettling to the patient who expects a definitive recommendation, price, and surgery date. Most plastic surgeons would be trying to sign her up by now and the patient may even judge me harshly in comparison to other plastic surgeons who do give them a price, a date, and reassurance of a *fabulous* result in less time than it takes to perform an EKG or chest X-ray. But temporary confusion will breed thoughtfulness in the patient who will ultimately become a well-informed candidate for surgery. The majority of patients will "get" it and appreciate the systematic and customized process of discovery and collaboration. If I still feel the patient is too deferential to me and lacks conviction in her own opinions, I'll tell her to think about it further and come back another day. *There is no reason to rush patients into surgery, especially if they don't know exactly what they want.* As much as it is joked about, there is no such thing as an emergency breast augmentation or emergency facelift.

In the next step of this process, taken either at the first visit or sometime in the future when she is more committed to the process, I will take the photographs. I invite her to bring in her own photographs to illustrate what she is looking for or, even more important, what she is *not* looking for. With elective cosmetic surgery, not doing harm or creating unhappiness is at least as important as attaining perceived perfection. It is better to gain a little than lose a lot.

The identification of the all-important point B may occur during the initial consultation. But more often than not, it takes a series of consultations where discussion often requires that compromises be made. These subsequent visits are the real working sessions when the patient and I collaborate to more clearly define point B. As we review options and make choices, the exact surgical maneuvers needed to achieve the goal become clearer. Emotional or physical goals are translated into anatomical goals. At some point, I will know precisely what will be done to what structure with what instrument to what degree. The patient will also have at least a basic understanding of the rationale for these maneuvers. Nothing I do is taken "off the rack." Each step in the surgical procedure will be rationalized and tailored to the patient's individual situation. If the personalized procedure fits an established model or prototype, fine. If not, so be it. There is nothing that says each patient should require the exact same steps as any other.

While I encourage patients to be as precise and specific as possible, I also caution about expecting perfection. Each maneuver has an inherent *margin of error,* some larger, some smaller than others. It is obvious that the more maneuvers performed, the greater the overall margin of error. It is like luggage and traveling by plane. The more legs of a trip and the more luggage you check in, the higher the chance you will lose some of your luggage. It pays to be as efficient as possible and do only what you need to do to be effective. Building the surgical blueprint step-by-step will ensure maximum efficiency.

The surgical plan at this point is entirely customized to the patient's individual desires and anatomy. What her girlfriend might have had may not apply. What she read online may have little relevance. What I did for the previous ninety-nine patients will not matter a great deal. It will be hard for some patients to screen out these voices in their heads and to focus on our small world. "But my girlfriend had..." they'll want to say. Forget your girlfriend. It's just the two of us.

At this point, we will be dealing with what I have referred to as the fifth dimension. Both the patient and I will have an understanding of her goals, the justification of the surgical game plan, and a sense of how successful the surgery will be. In addition, besides knowing the risks and complications of the surgery, the patient and I will be aware of the reasons for having options while in surgery and how I will be making decisions and choosing options. Sometimes there will be a fork in the road. And in anticipation of this, paraphrasing Yogi Berra, I will be able to take it (i.e., the correct path).

At some point, it will be important to consult with other doctors to assess the appropriateness, timing, and safety of a cosmetic procedure. In all but the simplest of procedures, I will require a medical clearance by a physician to ensure the health of the patients and be sure that everything necessary is done to optimize their medical condition and to minimize risk. This process might require blood tests, radiological tests, cardiac screening tests, mammograms, and urinalysis. Results of these tests may require revision of the surgical plan. A questionable mammogram may require postponement of breast surgery. Undetected anemia may demand a hematological workup or, in rare instances, pre-operative transfusion. Nearly every female of childbearing age will be asked to undergo a pregnancy test for obvious reasons. No one likes to be fooled into thinking that unthinkable things can't happen. They can.

Once my patient and I go through the doors of the surgical suite, it will be as collaborators, co-designers of the surgery. It is as if we are married. It is also at this point when her trust in me will help get her to point B in the safest way possible. When the patient is asleep, she is truly in my hands. It doesn't matter whether I am in scrubs to save life or limb, or to "merely" give quality of life. My path to the endpoint as determined by the fifth dimension will be quite clear, if not predictable and assured. If I need to innovate, it will have a rationale basis. If I need to modify, it will come by careful analysis. If I need to compromise, it will be in favor of the patient's desire and safety. Like any journey through life, uncertainties and vicissitudes of surgery will demand that I be able to think for, and act on behalf of, my patient. It is all about what she wants, not what I want her to want. It is in the operating room where all that preparation and discussion will pay off.

Now it might require compromises on both my part and my patient's to reach this point. Knowing that one can rarely, if ever, get something, let alone everything, for nothing, what the patient is willing to give up will determine what I end up doing as much as what she wants. For my part, I have to be willing to give up the patient if we do not reach the understanding of the fifth dimension. I truly believe patients must earn the right and privilege to risk their normal and healthy life and body for a "better" normal and healthy life and body. My practice and philosophy is not one of surgery on demand. I don't care if they are a celebrity or not. I take my job too seriously. If I don't comprehend what they see or what they want, or if they cannot accept limitations of the possibilities, we may part ways. My patient and I must be comfortable with all of our decisions and I must be confident in what the goals are as much as in my ability to perform the surgical maneuvers to reach those goals. In the end, the ordeal of the preparations should pay off in a safe and successful surgery.

After surgery, I follow a patient at regular intervals, usually within the first few days to change bandages or remove sutures. Then I see her every week for the first three weeks, at six weeks, three months, six months, and yearly. During this phase of recovery, I try to restrain her from making judgments since I know that what she sees is still changing, both physically and in her emotional response. The important thing for me is to manage her tissues as they heal but also maintain both of us in a positive state of mind in the face of pain, anxiety, uncertainty, and even possible disappointment. The goal in the end is for my patient to be in a better state of mind and body while accepting whatever imperfections may be present. The ordeal that I have put my patient through will ensure the highest probability of safety and satisfaction for both of us. It is an investment in my patient's future happiness and quality life. That's what cosmetic surgery is all about. And that is the truth.

CHAPTER 16:

THE TWELVE SACRED KNOW-NO'S OF COSMETIC PLASTIC SURGERY

* * *

1. Know Thy Past.
2. Know Thyself.
3. Know What You Can Risk.
4. Know What Makes You Happy and Where You Are Going.
5. Know What Makes You Unhappy and Where You Don't Want to Go.
6. Know How to Express Yourself.
7. No Lying.
8. Know Your Value (And That You Are Valuable).
9. Know Your Surgeon (Like Your Spouse).
10. No Negatives.
11. Know the Whys, Whats, and Hows of Your Surgery.
12. Know That Life Is Not Perfect.

1. Know Thy Past

The first thing a doctor does when he consults a patient is take a history. The history is critical for establishing a diagnosis and is often the only piece of information a doctor needs. Even in the not-so-distant past, before the advent of advanced diagnostic radiology and laboratory pathology, a careful history may have led to a nearly foolproof, so-called classic description of a very specific disease process that might apply to the majority of the afflicted patients. That is why they are called "classic." Tuberculosis, diabetes, myocardial infarction, and appendicitis all have classic histories.

There is an art to taking a history, especially when it is not so classic. It often requires both a detective-like mind trying to weave bits and pieces of facts into a comprehensive and logical story (as done so well by forensic pathologists). It also requires a sensitive and sympathetic soul to coax information that is sometimes not easily forthcoming from a reluctant, embarrassed, or emotional human being (as is imperative of a skilled psychologist). It is often lamented by old-time physicians (I suppose to some extent this makes me one) that the art and technique of taking a good history has been supplanted by all the diagnostic technology modern physicians have at their disposal. It also accounts for much of the increase in medical care cost since circumventing the availability of such technology in favor of pure history-taking and physical examination risks liability if you are wrong.

Once, while I was quizzing a third-year medical student about what to do with an accident victim complaining of abdominal pain, he replied, "Get a CT scan."

"Don't you want to do a history and physical exam first?" I replied.

In cosmetic surgery, the patient is often concerned about a facial or body appearance that has an immediate impact on her self-image. It is no different than the "complaint" a sick patient has who seeks necessary medical treatment. "My stomach hurts." "I have a runny nose." "I felt a lump." "My breasts are too saggy." "I don't like these bulges." The prospective patient or the surgeon may not devote much attention to the *history* of these complaints. It is the *here and now* that is of foremost important and one feels driven to *just fix the problem.* The patient may not think too much about the history of her large, sagging breasts (although when asked, she'll know), or the rate of temporal changes of her face, or, in the case of previous surgery, the specific details of each procedure. She simply wants to "fix" or "improve" the body part.

A good plastic surgeon will spend a great deal of time just talking to the patient and an attentive patient will be able to provide important information about his or her past. Each bit of datum may provide insight into how the patient's anatomy has changed (crucial to know how to "fix" the problem) or how the patient felt along the path to his or her present state (crucial to gauge how they will react psycho-emotionally to physical change or what will "improve" the look). We all have a past that has a lot to do with our present. Not exploring the past or focusing on the three-dimensional anatomy to the exclusion of the fourth-dimensional change in the anatomy risks misdiagnosing the "complaint." The appropriate solution that will produce the desired psycho-emotional effect of the patient might be miscalculated; the more information, the better. Often it is the change, or lack of it, from the patient's past to their present that causes them unhappiness. Unfortunately in this procedure-based era of medicine with a premium on quick solutions, taking a history doesn't pay very well and both doctor and patient can get used to taking shortcuts.

The most obvious example of this concept is in body contouring. When a patient walks into the office, disrobes, and points to bulging hips or protruding abdomen, rather than salivate giddily over the prospects of suctioning the thick fat she is grasping in her hands or of excising the excess skin she flips from side to side, I realize that a meticulous history of these areas might well reveal important details. Certain bulges will go away when she is more fit and toned. Here she might be able to significantly improve her look with a more rigorous attention to diet and exercise without assuming the risks of surgery. Perhaps she always had excess fat and skin even as a young adult. Surgery might then need to be customized in order not to return her to her past appearance or it might be incapable of producing a desired result because of her baseline natural state. If she is never the same weight for more than a few months at a time, the patient may not be a good surgical candidate at all.

The history of a patient's large breasts is important in determining how much is possibly hormonally related (as the size of a breast changes with puberty, pregnancy, breast-feeding, and menopause) and how much is related to body weight. It may also be helpful in estimating what size and shape is acceptable to the patient if she has traveled through varying sizes and shapes during her formative or reproductive years. In fact, with pregnancy and breast-feeding, a woman may travel from A-cup to D-cup and all the way back. This historical information will assist a keen surgeon in his or her choice of technique. I often have the patient bring in the bra she might have worn when she was her more voluptuous figure.

The past history is even more important when contemplating surgery on patients who have already had previous cosmetic surgical procedures—a common situation. Many breast implant patients (as many as 70 percent over the first decade after surgery) go through more than one procedure, either by necessity, as in leakage, displacement, or hardening, or by choice, as when they desire a change in size, type of implant, or secondary procedures like lifts. Knowing what occurred along the way may help a surgeon determine what has a good possibility of succeeding (or of failing). For a surgeon, repeating an operation that was well performed but turned out unacceptable is courting repeat failure. It is quite astonishing that many patients just do not know what their surgeon did to their bodies. Either they were not told, did not ask, forgot, or, for whatever reason, put it out of their mind. Most don't have records of their surgeries and rely on their surgeons to keep them, not realizing that records do not need to be, and usually are not, kept indefinitely. Secondary surgeries often occur many years after the first, beyond the time that records legally need to be maintained and certainly beyond the long-term memory retention of even the most brilliant surgeons.

In a common scenario, I had a patient who had saline breast implants placed by another surgeon a decade prior. One of the implants had deflated and required replacement. She had no records and the surgeon had since left practice. She stated that she thought the implants were 270 cc and smooth. Having no proof, I went through my usual measurements and determined that a certain implant of about 300 to 330 cc was appropriate because she wanted to be slightly larger. At surgery, it was discovered that she instead had 375-cc textured implants and was quite unhappy that the 360-cc implants we ended up using were actually smaller than what we took out. I was happy that her breasts looked quite like what was described as her goal pre-operatively. But trying to explain how the dimensional approach has supplanted the pure volumetric standard of years past didn't seem to appease her. What should have been a happy outcome was marred by a fixation on a number and by a lack of memory or record regarding her past surgery.

Knowing a patient's past can also help a doctor by avoiding doomed surgeries as well as selecting appropriate ones. The rare patient who desires or requires a second breast reduction can be in jeopardy of losing her nipple because of altered blood supply if technical details of the first operation are not known. Patients who travel from doctor to doctor seeking better and better results, but who become less and less satisfied, are especially risky candidates. The problem here is that these patients are more likely to hide their past experiences, distort or not remember the facts of their treatment, or entice doctors with exuberant praise or emotional lamentations in the hopes of persuading them to render further treatment. Unfortunately, some well-meaning and suffering patients who truly need a compassionate and talented surgeon may be swept under the rug of prejudgment and presumption.

The take-home message: If you do not know your past, your surgeon is at a disadvantage. If your surgeon does not ask you about your past, you may be at a disadvantage. Bottom line: **Know your past.**

2. Know Thyself

Of all know-no's, this is the most important and the most all-encompassing. It is so important to life that it was the central theme of my father's sermon, or toast, to me at my wedding. By now it must be evident that knowing who you are as the patient, as well as my knowing who I am as the surgeon, is crucial to an optimal outcome. It is not that you can't be satisfied with results if you don't heed this advice or go into surgery with blind devotion; after all, random play at the lottery, craps, and love can win you the jackpot. Even dart-throwing amateur stock-pickers, as well as Raven, a live monkey of the fabled MonkeyDex of Wall Street, can pick stocks that beat the pros about 40 percent of the time.

However, the pursuit of plastic surgery is really the *purposeful* pursuit of happiness. Unlike golf, where being lucky is sporadically better than being good, cosmetic surgery requires more careful planning, knowledge, and execution than fortuitous luck. Happiness can be found in self-confidence, in acceptance, in feeling attractive, in feeling special, in being able to wear normal or fashionable clothes. Cosmetic surgery is merely a vehicle to achieve these goals with the expectation of becoming *happier* in its broadest sense. While this seems quite obvious, it is surprising to talk to patients who either have little idea of what will make them happy, only that they are indeed *un*happy.

They are so willing to relinquish their definitions of happiness to those of a stranger in the hopes that the stranger behind the mask wielding a #20 saber blade knows something about what will make them happy more than they themselves do. It is a calculated risk and a measured roll of the dice that patients take every day.

As one matures, it becomes more apparent who you are. It doesn't mean you are aware of it or can define it or are happy with it. But there is, with exceptions of course, a pattern of behavior and choice that makes each person unique. Young teenagers and adults may think they know who they are, and they might, but often it is, in reality, just immature braggadocio or development-related insecurity. That is why one must be cautious in performing cosmetic surgery on teenagers. It is not uncommon to hear patients come back later on in life regretting the surgery they had, or were "forced" to have by their parents, as a teenager or young adult. Of course, many will also look at their surgery as life-saving. The challenge is to know who knows herself and who doesn't.

Age itself is not an antidote to immaturity and certainly not to unhappiness or discontent. We all know adults who are immature. Some might even think people who get cosmetic surgery are, by definition, immature. Rather, it is the knowing of what will make one happy that is an ideal prerequisite, even if what will make one happy is considered immature (or example, getting a tattoo or body ring or even breast implants). Then it is up to the surgeon to debate and negotiate the reasonableness or the safety of the request. Here, we are concerned mainly about *individual, not societal,* happiness and safety.

The irony is that the patient who knows who she is may be harder to "work" with if the doctor is paternalistic (sort of like having an authoritative parent negotiating with a headstrong teenager). She will later often complain to another doctor that the first doctor never listened to her. It is much easier to not ask the patient or teenager and just do what you, the surgeon or parent, think is right or good; the easiest patient to operate on is the unconscious patient. On the other hand, a collaborative surgeon, like me, finds it a delight to consult with an insightful and introspective patient. Here, there is give-and-take, a negotiation, and a final denouement that can feel like a satisfying major triad chord at the end of an interminable Beethoven coda.

One important aspect to knowing oneself is being able to feel confident going against conventional wisdom and to make decisions independent of others. Today's society is constantly flooded with images and stories that influence people and how they live, whether it be a certain style, a particular look, the size of breasts, or what is considered healthy, hip, or attractive. The herd mentality and the desire for people to belong or fit in, especially the young and insecure, can place heavy pressure on patients to do what is in vogue, and that includes trendy cosmetic procedures. I am constantly on the lookout for the individuality of people and an indication that a person knows herself well enough to desire something *independent of the opinion of others*. A plastic surgeon's operating table is the last place you'd want to see a factory assembly line. Even a patient's decision not to have surgery can be a good thing, for that patient. Being able to reject cosmetic surgery is just as important, valid, and self-affirming as committing to cosmetic surgery.

In determining when a patient is an appropriate candidate for body-contouring procedures, I apply my test of a healthy, stable lifestyle. I have confidence that a good patient knows herself well enough that she knows when she is not putting in a full effort to achieve a healthy, stable lifestyle. She knows whether her diet can be improved and whether her exercise routine needs to be increased. She knows how easy or hard it might be to maintain a certain weight and knows the things that will prevent her from attaining a certain lifestyle. All this self-knowledge helps guide decision-making and the collaboration with a surgeon towards a safe, smart, successful outcome.

When you sign up for cosmetic surgery, **know who you are.**

3. Know What You Can Risk

If this sounds like a gambling tip, it is! We all know the caveats with going to Las Vegas or investing in stocks: Know what you can lose and stick with it. Don't throw good money after bad. Investing is all about limiting downside risks. You can lose money faster than you can make it. The performance of a portfolio is determined not by your winners, but by your losers. We've all been there: hoping for the best, ignoring the worst, and kicking ourselves when it happens.

The same is true for cosmetic surgery. So much emphasis is on what a patient desires and what a doctor can or will do that little time or thought is spent on what one can lose or what complication or negative side effect can occur. All the players in this scene are focused on getting through the operating room doors. The problem is that no procedure has zero risk, no patient thinks complications will happen to her, and few surgeons want to proactively say things that will discourage patients from having a surgery that might, indeed, make them happier. That is why the informed consent, the document that is usually explained to patients by someone other than the doctor and that contains a dizzying array of scary medical terms and descriptive events, is so important. While these potential side effects and complications are glossed over by most patients, perhaps not even read in its entirety, and most likely forgotten twenty-four hours later, they are the main cause for producing *un*happiness, rather than happiness.

We assume that patients know that surgery is not risk-free. They may be uninformed as to *specific* risks but they are not naïve as to presume *zero* risks. The challenge to the patient is to know how to prioritize these risks and decide which are acceptable to them and which are not. Risks are not shortcomings you have to accept. They are known trade-offs or undesirable outcomes that will occur to someone and that patients and surgeons need to manage.

A recent patient with a rather simple problem came to see me. He had a persistent, firm swelling on his forehead that was cosmetically undesirable and determined to be related to a blunt trauma five years ago. I was prepared to perform the excision (possibly including some overgrowth of bone) from an incision behind his hairline so the scar could be hidden. Upon being presented with the alternative of an incision directly over the lump that would in fact make my job easier, he, against his mother's preference, stated he preferred the scar be placed directly over the mass in a forehead crease despite the risk that this scar might be more visible than the other and that it might not heal perfectly. He obviously could tolerate the risk of having a visible scar on his forehead. Others might not.

Another common example is in breast augmentation. While there are advantages and disadvantages to using saline or silicone gel implants, the number one reason one might want to use a silicone gel breast implant is that when it works as intended, it feels more natural than a saline implant. If it weren't for the softness, silicone gel implants wouldn't even be on the market. Anyone who chooses silicone gel over saline must be willing to accept all of the associated risks of leakage and increased incidence and degree of capsular contracture or hardening. The fact that they do choose this implant means they willingly accept these risks. This includes the not insubstantial costs of repeat surgery. This post-surgical financial risk is largely ignored as the affordability of initial cosmetic surgery, through competition and credit financing, has successfully revolutionized the field from a luxury expenditure for the rich and famous to a matter of simple capital allocation or monthly budgeting for the everyday, normal person. But just like the devastating effects of a credit or mortgage crunch, not knowing what one can afford or risk beyond just the short term is ill-advised. Imagine how upset you would be if you were presented with another bill a few years later because one of the known risks of leakage, hardening, or displacement had occurred and you hadn't fully accepted those risks. That is also one of the misinterpretations of statistical risks; even though an individual risk is statistically uncommon, such as a one percent risk of infection, when it actually does happen to a patient, your number has been called and you have to be able to deal with it a hundred percent.

Risk-taking involves the possibility of accepting something undesirable or giving up something desirable. A scar is obvious. Loss of hair or sensation is common. Even losing one's life is discussed and contemplated. Some patients have had to cancel trips and cruises because of post-operative complications. That is why I advise giving plenty of time to recover, even without a complication, before you need to commit to a social event. Your body does not care what your social calendar looks like, even though many patients have cosmetic surgery specifically for a social event like a reunion or wedding.

Assuming a risk also involves an emotional investment. How many think they might lose a partner? There can be tremendous strain on a relationship because of the psycho-emotional changes that may or may not occur and this is one of the reasons it is important to explore the problems and strengths of a patient's interpersonal relationships. I had one couple come in contemplating breast surgery for the wife. After a number of office visits, it was clear that they had a strained marriage and the proposed surgery magnified the strain and intrinsic disagreements in their relationship. The wife never went through the surgery and a half a decade later, the husband brought in his new wife for a similar consultation. A similar situation must have existed since that wife also did not go through with surgery.

One might be willing to risk a scar or life or limb, but can you risk the anxiety of worrying about your surgical results? I had one patient who despite reviewing all the statistics and carefully choosing to have silicone gel implants for her breast augmentation just could not adapt to the possibility of her implants leaking. She worried that every little unusual sensation meant her implant had ruptured. This placed a strain on her relationship with her husband and she ended up exchanging them for saline implants.

When changing appearances, there is a risk that a patient may feel even more self-conscious (for instance, a woman who wants to have breast enlargement but doesn't want any of her partners to know) or may be unable to feel comfortable in her new skin. I have seen a number of patients, particularly males operated on by other surgeons, who wanted their rhinoplasty results reversed. Now some of these situations may be the result of poor results in less than ideal candidates, but that is exactly the problem. Results cannot be guaranteed, complications cannot be eliminated, and psycho-emotional response cannot be predicted. You have to know what risks you can accept.

4. Know What Makes You Happy and Where You Are Going

This recommendation seems so obvious since patients usually come into the office focused on a particular anatomical area. However, often they are blinded by their discontent with that bodily feature. That is, it is more that they are unhappy with a certain look than they are desirous of a particular new one. While this is not universal, it is common enough that it is important to realize that not all patients know what will make them happy; they just know what is making them *un*happy. Part of the dilemma for the patients is that they may feel less responsible for choosing a result because they do not know what is possible. They have a misconception, in large part perpetuated by the media and advertising, that they have to accept a certain look. "What will I look like after a facelift?" is a common question.

I constantly struggle with patients to get them to clearly define their specific goals and, even more so, not to rely entirely on my opinion. My mentor, D. Ralph Millard, Jr., M.D., devoted a small chapter in his tome, *Principlization of Plastic Surgery*, to the principle, "Have a Goal and a Dream." While much of his emphasis was on the plastic surgeon requiring a specific target, dedication, persistence, and concentration to attain a surgical result, this principle is even more important for the patient. The plastic surgeon is assumed to possess these qualities because of training, but the patient is the final arbiter of the surgical endeavor. If he or she doesn't know what the goal is and what he or she wants, how can the plastic surgeon succeed?

Success in surgery is not unlike success in life. You can occasionally stumble on success in individual circumstances, but I wouldn't advise relying on stumbling to get you through life or surgery. Patients must put in effort and do their homework as much as the plastic surgeons. In fact, plastic surgeons should give patients homework that defines their goals. As in acquiring directions to reach a particular destination, the patient's individual goals should produce a surgical and mental map for the plastic surgeon. The patient's task is a delicate balance of expecting something but not too much, of being as specific as possible without being unrealistically specific, and of having a goal without clinging uncompromisingly to that single goal.

An example of this is found in abdominoplasty surgery. An abdominoplasty is really a generic term that does not refer to a specific procedure, although most patients may not understand that. Generally speaking, it refers to surgical contouring of the torso involving tightening of the abdominal muscles and excision of fat and skin. There are multiple variations and categorizations of these variations based on patterns of abdominal shape and anatomical deformities. In reality, decisions must be made regarding various components of the operation: where to place the resulting scar; how long to make the scar; how much, if any, skin should be removed and from where; how and to what extent fat should be removed; relative importance of removing damaged skin with stretch marks that can affect the position of the scar; whether or not to move the belly button (umbilicus) and how; how and to what degree muscles should be tightened. When patients know specifically what they want to change, what they want to get rid of, what they want to keep, and what they ultimately want to look like, a very specific abdominoplasty can be performed. But the patient might need to make specific choices that demand compromises. If she wants all the stretch marks gone, the scar might have to be higher. If she wants the scar to be as low as possible, she might not be able to have a full abdominoplasty without a second scar. If she wants the tightest and thinnest abdomen possible, she might have to do two operations in stages. The desire determines the technique, not the other way around.

Many people are unhappy with their working lives.[10] Half of all employed people are dissatisfied with their

10 I Can't Get No...Job Satisfaction, That is, *The Conference Board*, January 2010

jobs with only about 20 percent of the satisfied employees being *very* satisfied. That is not the main problem, though. The main problem is that many people do not know what *will* make them happy and satisfied. They are constantly searching. They never find their "calling." They get trapped in a passionless job.

Unhappiness starts early. Even by college, many students find themselves unhappy. When I went to college in the early 1970s, one of the most popular courses at Harvard was Economics 10. It required two large auditoriums to accommodate over one thousand students, more than half the entering freshman class. Now it is a course on happiness called "Positive Psychology" taught by Tal Ben-Sharer, who stresses certain general principles, including the idea that happiness requires both pleasure and meaning, obvious when one thinks about having fun with loved ones versus strangers. He also emphasizes the need to find deep personal meaning in things, perhaps such as cosmetic surgery, since even though there is a connection between the body (i.e., breast, nose, or face) and the mind, happiness is more a state of mind.

As a patient, you need to get what you want out of cosmetic surgery or else there is no point in getting it and you can only get what you want if you know what you want. You won't find vegetables while browsing in the meat department.

5. Know What Makes You Unhappy and Where You Don't Want to Go

This is a corollary to Know-No numbers 3 and 4. As much as it is important for a plastic surgeon to know how to get to where he wants to go based on what the patient desires, it is just as important to know what *not* to do because of where the patient *doesn't* want to go. Some of the unhappiest patients are those who end up with complication-free results that just aren't what they wanted or imagined. It is not that the surgeon did a poor operation, but that perhaps he did the "wrong" one for that patient or made judgments not aligned with the patient's individual desires. The result might have been perfectly acceptable, even fantastic, but for a different patient. The fault can almost always be traced back to lack of communication between the surgeon and the patient.

By lack of communication, I mean exactly that—it is not a miscommunication, or a misunderstanding, or a misinterpretation; it is a *lack* of communication. The conversation of what a patient *does not want* never takes place. The ideal patient will state exactly what she does not want. "I don't want a pulled look." "I don't want to look done." "I don't want the deer-frozen-in-the-headlights look." "I don't want the two-grapefruits-stuck-on-my-chest look." "I don't want to be too perky." Even the impossible request, "I don't want any scars" is an important one to make because it establishes the remote likelihood of success and patient happiness because virtually all surgeries will end up having scars. The surgeon will need a more realistic expectation from the patient. Some omissions may be shortsighted on the surgeon's part, but a patient should not put herself in the position after surgery of having to say, "I should have told the doctor I didn't want…"

By the same token, a patient who encounters a surgeon who takes offense at hearing what the patient will not tolerate might not have a surgical result customized to his or her desires. That same surgeon is likely not to take seriously the patients' communication of what they do want. To me, any information that gives a direction to achieve a patient's end result is helpful. I will often pose hypothetical situations so that I can make an informative decision about what a patient will or won't accept.

One example is prioritizing surgical procedures. Many patients will opt to undergo multiple procedures simultaneously. I then ask, "Which procedure, if not done, would make you most unhappy?" By finding out which procedure is most important and which ones they definitely want to get or definitely will not miss, I can prioritize the intra-operative order in case the surgery needs to be curtailed. I am always thinking about patient safety.

Another example is in determining breast size. Sometimes, exact size cannot be predicted precisely since it involves multiple dimensions and variables (volume, width, projection, shape, natural breast, pliability of soft tissues, size of implant relative to final breast, and chest anatomy). I always have a few choices of breast implant sizes available. I will ask a patient what will make her unhappier: having breasts that are larger or ones that are smaller than expected. I ask the same type of question with lifts or reductions: What will make you *more* unhappy—having breasts with less shape or more scars? Or abdominoplasties: What will make you *more* unhappy—skin that is still loose or stretch marks that are still present? I also stress that it is often more helpful to bring in pictures of breasts they do not like: too large, too small, too wide, too much cleavage, etc., etc.

Determining which road the patient is less willing to travel down can be of tremendous value in making specific surgical decisions. Men certainly appreciate the directness of women telling them what will make them unhappy as opposed to trying to guess what might make them happy. From child to student to law-abiding adult citizen, we often understand don'ts better than do's.

6. Know How to Express Yourself

I know this may sound like a touchy-feely, New Age thing, but it is crucially important. It is usually the doctor who is being criticized for a lack of expressing himself, or failure of communicating, of being too clinical, or not explaining things enough in understandable layman's term. Certainly a majority of malpractice lawsuits occur because of breakdown in communication either between doctor and doctor, or doctor and patient. When a doctor does possess the unique quality of being able to explain a disease or a situation or a treatment to a patient in a simple, non-condescending manner, patients not only appreciate it but usually think even more highly of the doctor as compassionate and caring. This will lead to more trust. When this communication does not occur, the patient feels confused, insignificant, and mistrustful.

The same is true for patient expression and communication. Medical care that is necessary often, rightfully or not, does not include the patient's feelings or preference. In fact, the dispassionate arm of medicine can sometimes override an individual's own desire. Certain urgent circumstances don't even need the patient to be conscious for treatment. In elective cosmetic surgery, the patient's feelings and preference are the *only* things that matter. Yet it is surprising when speaking to patients who had complications or were unhappy with their results how often they admitted that they failed to express exactly what they wanted and how they felt to the doctor. Whether they cowered like students in front of their intimidating professor, took for granted that their surgeon "knew" what they wanted, or failed to formulate their own desires, they all lead to failure of self-expression.

It is the responsibility of the patient to care enough about her own health and goals. When a patient isn't given the opportunity by her surgeon to express herself, she might rethink about the appropriateness of that surgeon for her. In any collaborative process, like any successful partnership, communication is a two-way street. Much of my focus in teaching plastic surgery residents is getting them to listen to their patients and to force or free their patients to express themselves in very specific terms. When designing a new face or body, it is not the time to be timid and silent, nor is it the time to resign yourself to a surgeon who won't allow you to **express yourself**.

7. No Lying

Once again, this seems self-evident. It is what parents teach their kids and what is expected of professionals like doctors. Yet patients will sometimes purposefully mislead plastic surgeons. I am not talking about a pathological behavior since that, by definition, cannot be easily controlled by a well-reasoning patient. Patients with Munchausen syndrome or body dysmorphism disorder have psychiatric reasons for being untruthful in order to gain sympathy or access to some desired treatment or medication. But perfectly healthy cosmetic patients can also color or subjugate the truth. Patients claim to be free of tobacco, alcohol, or drugs in order to proceed with cosmetic surgery. Patients deny having had previous procedures, especially rhinoplasty, for fear of being rejected for having too much surgery or being judged as frivolous or vain. Patients misguide their surgeon about their activities or behavior before or after surgery to mask their own irresponsibility.

Patients need to be reminded that the ultimate responsibility of the plastic surgeon should be patient safety because the surgery itself is unnecessary. No gain in one's appearance is worth a terrible complication. Complications are unexpected and undesirable things that can happen to complicate a disease or treatment. By definition, a complication complicates the situation. Both patient and doctor should do everything to reduce the risk of a complication even though they cannot eliminate it. Lying, however a patient justifies it, can produce decisions that, because not founded on fact and truth, lead to real complications. Lying about cigarette smoking can lead to devastating tissue necrosis. Lying about alcohol and drugs can lead to withdrawal symptoms, seizures, and cross-reactions with anesthetic and other medicinal agents. Lying about past surgeries can lead to performing the wrong surgery, traumatizing marginally healthy tissues, or repeating surgeries that have already failed. In almost every situation, while not always leading to dire consequences, lying does nothing to advance patient safety and may directly reduce patient safety.

In short, **lying hurts**. If you don't want the doctor to lie to you, don't lie to the doctor, no matter what you believe you have to gain.

8. Know Your Value (and That You Are Valuable)

Again, this sounds like a self-evident, sentimental catchphrase for the new millennium. Most women who read any of the current magazines intended for the modern woman or listen to any of the talk shows directed toward projecting a positive image of women will be familiar with the message of empowerment. The message applies equally to men. Yet it is an ambiguous message with internal contradictions that can be interpreted in diametrically opposed ways.

On the one hand, there is a challenge for individuals to be content and to accept oneself for who one is, whether it be that one is independent-thinking, overweight, underweight, small-busted, voluptuous, career-oriented, kitchen-bound, same-sex oriented, or transgender-minded. On the other hand, there is also a liberating clarion call of encouraging women in particular to pursue self-improvement, to break glass ceilings, to challenge men on their turf, to not settle for the status quo. While the actions one takes because of these points of view may be different, the underlying assumption is similar; *no person is absent of value.* Knowing you have value will assist in making decisions. Having value does not mean one has to be complacent with that value. Having self-esteem and being in search of self-improvement are not mutually exclusive states.

Patients will often seek out cosmetic surgery because they feel handicapped, or inferior, or alienated, or perhaps embarrassed. Healthy self-esteem is at stake and may be virtually non-existent in some patients. A patient can see improvement through plastic surgery as a solution, a way out, an escape. While seemingly a positive step, and not denying that it may in fact be a positive action, getting cosmetic surgery while in the wrong frame of mind can produce a potentially harmful effect; the surgery may not produce a desired physical change and any perceived shortcoming or resulting complication or unwanted side effect may jeopardize what little value a patient sees in his- or herself to begin with. These patients are on shaky ground at the outset.

The answer to this predicament is either to possess sufficient self-confidence and self-worth *prior to* surgery such that the foundation on which a patient stands while going through surgery is firm and well-grounded, or to acknowledge real value in oneself such that the plastic surgery one thinks is the answer no longer seems that desperately critical but becomes merely additive to one's life. It is a delicate balance of possessing just enough perceived need and desire to undergo elective cosmetic surgery while not being overly dependent on that need and desire. Self-valued patients usually mean emotionally healthy patients. Just as in life, a person who sees value in herself and who is supported by her own ego will have a more realistic attitude and will be more able to tolerate the possible shortcomings inherent in all surgery. **Find your value.**

9. Know Your Surgeon (Like Your Spouse)

In any collaborative endeavor, like cosmetic surgery, trust is imperative. While it might seem that knowing and trusting are contradictory (that is, you need not rely on trust if you know, and if you lack knowledge then you need to trust), they are really *inter*dependent and not mutually exclusive. While trust is applied to things one cannot or does not know, it is dependent to some extent on what knowledge one does have. Complete trust can be the result of the belief in something without any verifiable or objective knowledge, as in trusting a stranger or God, or it can be a result of having the maximum amount of knowledge about what is verifiable, as in trusting that a ball will bounce back from the ground if you drop it from your hand.

I like to draw parallels between the surgeon-patient relationship and an interpersonal relationship since the issue of trust is the same. In marriages or relationships arranged by others in certain cultures or societies, there is the ultimate need for trust because there is no knowledge. The only knowledge that exists is between the partners and the go-between; perhaps they know (and trust) the matchmaker or their parents. On the other hand, once you are with someone for a long time, you build a fund of knowledge that, while never absolutely foolproof, reduces the need for trust because you "know." Of course, this assumes that what you know is truly the truth and not a façade. In action based on trust, there is, however small, a "leap of faith"; the more you know, the shorter that leap, and the more predictable the relationship.

When I hear a patient is having surgery by a doctor about whom she knows very little and has met only once for a few minutes, I wonder where that trust comes from. I suppose that is the definition of "blind" trust. Assuming there will always be a requirement of, and belief in, the benefit of minimizing this leap of faith, it stands to reason logically that the more knowledge you have of the person doing your surgery, the less you need to rely on "blind" trust. This is good. No one wants "blind" and "surgery" to be used in the same sentence. It's almost like putting "Hollywood" and "marriage" together. Now I am not only talking about medical knowledge, experience, or education. You would ideally like to know a little more about the person you are going to marry than what job he or she has, how much he or she earns, what kind of car he or she drives, or what neighborhood he or she lives in. You want to know what kind of person he or she is. Is he patient, kind, compassionate, generous, forgiving, spiritual, athletic, passionate, interesting, ambitious, honest, etc., etc., etc.? Will she be dependable, resilient, supportive, industrious, unselfish, thoughtful, etc., etc., etc.? What is his or her philosophy of life?

Now, of course I do not really mean to say that *all* this knowledge is pertinent to a cosmetic surgical outcome. But *some* of it *may* be. What I tell my patients is that when there is money in the bank, the kids are fine, and everyone is healthy, then all is well and everyone is happy. The real question is what happens when the money runs low, the kids are in trouble, and some catastrophe hits? What kind of person is your partner? Is the relationship strong enough to endure? Can two people find common ground and trust each other to find solutions? Or will mistrust, blame, self-interest, and uncertainty rule the day? I don't worry about the successes, because they make people happy. I worry about the failures, because they do not. The only way you can secure the relationship, overcome failures, and minimize blind trust is to know as much as you can about your partner, in this case, the plastic surgeon. Lacking any knowledge, trusting then becomes mere guessing.

This is especially true in today's world of Internet information and advertising. The best patients have

always been, and still are, those that have been personally referred by a medical colleague, a friend or family
member, or a former patient, all of whom essentially
act as the trusted matchmaker. The same is true for
plastic surgeons. As follows the world-is-flat theory of
Thomas Friedman, advertising, specifically Internet
advertising, levels the playfield, but also makes it
harder to distinguish quality of plastic surgeons. We
all start to look the same in pixels.

Learn about, and get to know, your plastic surgeon
because there is such a thing as being *too* trusting.
After all, a good surgeon is going to learn as much as
possible about you; he is also looking for the "good
partner."

10. No Negatives

Since having cosmetic surgery is like getting married, it is logical that this Know-No follows Know-No
number 9. There is a certain amount of knowledge
you must have about your surgeon and your surgeon
must have about you. I've argued that there is a varying degree of trust that exists between all parties. You
shouldn't have too many negative thoughts about
the process upon which you are about to embark. Of
course, you have to expect some doubt and uncertainty to creep into your head and private conversations. After all, you don't want to be naïve about the
journey; surgery is not like getting a haircut. The most
common emotions expressed by patients in the pre-
operative room are the conflicting emotions of excitement and fear or anticipation and anxiety or happiness
and nervousness. Sounds like most pre-matrimonial
butterflies.

Everyone knows half of the marriages end in divorce, and even more after a second marriage. Complications from surgery are similar. Everyone knows, or should know, that complications exist. As with divorce, hopefully you want to do everything possible to minimize complications. Most of what I have tried to write about is directed towards achieving a successful surgery and minimizing complications.

There are benefits to having an enthusiastic attitude, a healthy physical and mental condition, and minimal stress. Going into surgery with a positive frame of mind means, and requires, that a patient is prepared and ready for the journey. This will mean that she will have asked, and have answered, the important questions to the degree that both plastic surgeon and patient are completely satisfied. There will be no lingering mysteries or second-guessing. There will be a confidence that both the patient and the plastic surgeon are meant for each other, dedicated to each other, respect each other, and have common goals. Not only is there an understanding that those goals are attainable, but also that, if for some reason they are not (as can happen), the plastic surgeon will be able to navigate the patient through the difficult times and that the patient will likewise stand by the plastic surgeon as his/her ally and protector. If there are negative thoughts about the surgeon's expertise or trustworthiness, or about one's choices, or about the operating room facility, or the financial arrangement, things can fall apart very quickly.

Having no negative thoughts is not only about banishing the inevitable negatives but also putting in the effort in the preparation such that negative thoughts cannot even exist. Performers like professional athletes work hard to attain positive attitude and visualization of success. When pro golfer Vijay Singh won the 2000 Masters, he credited his son for putting his mind in the correct frame for success with a note on his bag saying, "Poppa, trust your swing"—a perfect example of incorporating the confidence of having the knowledge of possessing a great swing with the staunch belief in the positive outcome of the unknown. The same is true in the performing arts. Music teachers and acting coaches are always trying to get performers to forget about the difficulty of technique or the fear of forgetting. **Once you start thinking you can't or shouldn't do something, you are finished.** The last thing you want your surgeon to hear while wheeling you into the operating room is, "I really don't know if…"

11. Know the Whys, Whats, and Hows of Your Surgery

I don't know how many times I have been surprised by what patients choose *not* to know about their cosmetic surgery. From not wanting to hear about complications to transferring responsibility of choice onto the shoulders of their surgeon, patients can adopt an attitude of "the less I know, the better for me." They are happy with the paternalistic style of medicine. They don't need to know why the computer works, just how to use it. They don't need to know what goes into a delicious dish, just if it tastes good to them. They don't want to learn how a car runs, just how to drive from A to B. The ironic thing is that all this information is readily available to them.

Medicine, and especially plastic surgery, has come directly to the consumer so that there is no need to be ignorant about anything that is being done to one's body. Taking responsibility for one's body will always make for a better patient. No surgeon should be reluctant to share with a patient the reasons he or she chooses to do things a certain way. When dealing with patients undergoing medically necessary treatment, patients are encouraged to learn as much as they can about their condition and available treatments. Doctors who do not adequately inform patients should be admonished. Lawsuits can easily arise from the lack of this information and education. It stands to reason that when seeking elective, cosmetic treatment, the requirement for knowledge should be even greater. Why do something to your body and face that you don't have to without full knowledge of what, why, and how?

I am quite wary of patients who do not ask important and probing questions or who do not challenge the explanations and reasons for surgical treatments. When patients do not need to take the risk of cosmetic surgery, it bothers me that they are cavalier about those risks. If they are too accepting of what I am planning to do, but do not understand what exactly is it I am planning to do, they may be pliable, but ignorant, patients. If there is a truly collaborative approach to their treatment, it gives me a reassuring sense that they are as fully informed, understanding of, and committed to their treatment as a layperson can be. It means that we have hopefully crossed all the t's and dotted all the i's and turned over as many rocks as we can think of. A good surgeon will appreciate the patient's interest and involvement. He will feel more secure in her knowledge of, and commitment to, the surgical process.

The old-fashioned approach of "don't ask, don't tell" just isn't hip today.

12. Know That Life Is Not Perfect

This pretty much sums up the state of one's personal universe and is as close to a truism as I can think of, even though it may be contrary to what a person wants to hear as she goes through her cosmetic surgery. While basking in the glittering life-improving glory of cosmetic surgery, a patient can lose sight of this concept. Some will seek perfection in themselves, their surgery, their surgeon, and their life. Disappointment will accompany any shortcoming in the pursuit of perfection and they, as well as their surgeons, can become entrapped in the vicious game of "Chasing the Imperfections." It is not so much that the grass is always greener in another pasture, but that whatever pasture one is in is just not green enough. A bigger and wider perspective is needed than the focused, sometimes myopic, viewpoint assumed by self-interested cosmetic patients. Managing expectations, preparing a patient for imperfection, being ready to accept certain improvements and not look back can save both patient and surgeon a lot of future grief. Being able to get a patient to see outside of herself will temper the, at times, seemingly justifiable tenacious grip of discontent.

I do not mean that self-interest is necessarily bad since that is predominantly the motivation from which cosmetic patients come. In fact, I have argued all along that it is *self*-interest, not *other*-interest, which must be the obligatory motivating factor. The caveat is that of self-interest at the *exclusion* of all other interest and perspective—vanity. Believe me, I have seen that happen to the most well-intended, rational patient.

Admittedly, I am guilty at times of creating this seemingly perfect world of attaining one's dreams. By taking the patient through this meticulous process of customization and individualization, I might project the image that anything is possible, that we can turn a sow's ear into a gold purse. In my forcing patients to be as specific and detailed as possible in their description of what they desire, they might paint themselves into the tight corner of high expectations. The journey of accomplishing a cosmetic change is like taking a trip from Los Angeles to Boston. I do not want them to end up in Miami or Dallas. Yet they might come to expect a specific room in a specific hotel and become grievously unhappy when they can't get the corner suite with the ocean view.

People, patients or not, can be unhappy with so many blessings in their pockets. I must constantly remind my patients as well as myself of the truth hiding behind the glitter and the mask. And the truth is: **Life and cosmetic surgery are not perfect, but both certainly can be beautiful.**

ABOUT THE AUTHOR

* * *

D r. Robin T.W. Yuan is a graduate of Harvard College and Harvard Medical School. A board-certified plastic surgeon in private practice, he is an attending surgeon at Cedars-Sinai Medical Center and an assistant clinical professor at UCLA School of Medicine.

Dr. Yuan has been named by his peers as one of L.A.'s "SuperDoctors" in cosmetic surgery and as one of "America's Top Doctors" by Castle Connelly Medical Publisher. He is listed in Marquis' *Who's Who in America* and *Who's Who in Science and Technology*. In addition, Dr. Yuan was one of the plastic surgeons chosen to be featured during the original season of ABC's *Extreme Makeover.*

He enjoys tennis, golf, writing, and playing the violin, among other activities. His first book, *Cheer Up, You're Only Half Dead (Reflections at Mid-life),* was published in 1996 and his other book, *The Skinny ... on Marriage: A Plastic Surgeon's Practical Guide,* is soon to be published. He lives in Beverly Hills with his son, Ryan, daughter, Robyn Nicole, and their Welsh Corgi, Blaze.